# TO DO'S

Safe People
~~Book~~
Kindle

Buy - Sleeping Pills - Matuxy
Clean Porch
Garage Sale
Oscar - Quote.
Patio Furniture
  2nd. Hand Store.

Pepinos

Cookies
Jugos
Ham / Pan
Kids Punch.
Bananas
Sandia
Spinich
Salad
Kale.
Tomatoes

String

of

Pearls

To Cotton

May my words help

you polish your

own pearls!

*(signature)*

# Also by JoAnna M. Lund

*The Healthy Exchanges Cookbook*

*HELP: The Healthy Exchanges Lifetime Plan*

*Cooking Healthy with a Man in Mind*

*Cooking Healthy with the Kids in Mind*

*Dessert Every Night!*

*Make a Joyful Table*

*The Diabetic's Healthy Exchanges Cookbook*

*The Strong Bones Healthy Exchanges Cookbook*

*The Arthritis Healthy Exchanges Cookbook*

*The Heart Smart Healthy Exchanges Cookbook*

*The Best of Healthy Exchanges Food Newsletter '92 Cookbook*

*Letters from the Heart*

*It's Not a Diet, It's a Way of Life* (audiotape)

# JoAnna M. Lund

*with*

*Barbara Alpert*

G. P. PUTNAM'S SONS

NEW YORK

# String

## of

# Pearls

Recipes for Living Well
in the Real World

G. P. Putnam's Sons
*Publishers Since 1838*
a member of
Penguin Putnam Inc.
375 Hudson Street
New York, NY 10014

Library of Congress Cataloging-in-Publication Data
Lund, JoAnna M.
String of pearls : recipes for living well in the real world /
JoAnna M. Lund with Barbara Alpert.
p.   cm.
ISBN 0-399-14654-7
1. Quality of life.   2. Change (Psychology).   I. Alpert, Barbara.   II. Title.
BF637.C5.L86      2000                  00-035639
613.2'5—dc21

Printed in the United States of America

1   3   5   7   9   10   8   6   4   2

This book is printed on acid-free paper. ∞

BOOK DESIGN BY AMANDA DEWEY

This book is dedicated to the loving memory of my parents, Jerome and Agnes McAndrews. While they are no longer with me, I know they are in Heaven watching as I apply the earthly talents I inherited from them to help others help themselves. Mom and Daddy wouldn't have it any other way. I share one of my mother's thoughtful poems that addresses this very subject:

### Thoughts to Live By

When a promise is made it should be kept;
    otherwise it could become a lie.
The good intentions we neglect to keep
    are accountable for when we die.
God gives all of us our own unique talents
    and He intends for them to be used.
For they are truly special gifts from Him
    that should not ever be abused.
Good examples will influence others
    in everything that we do and say.
Like a mirror they reflect into our soul,
    to spread happiness along the way.

—*Agnes Carrington McAndrews*

# Acknowledgments

For helping me polish my pearls to share with you, I want to thank:

*John Duff and Susan Petersen Kennedy*—They saw that I had more to share than just recipes and asked me to commit to paper the ideas that I talk about in person.

*Barbara Alpert*—She has the ability to take my words, both written and spoken, and make them more than the sum of their parts. Together, we both become better.

*Cliff Lund*—He's heard me share what I've learned on my own personal journey toward good health and self-acceptance at least a thousand times. But whenever he drives me to another speaking engagement, he gives me the courage and support to share it all over again.

*God*—When I prayed for the guidance to stop dieting and start living healthier, I never dreamed He would bless me with talents in my middle years. Along with that blessing comes a responsibility to share with others what I've learned.

# Contents

Introduction     *1*

Learning to Accept What You Cannot Change     *15*

Listening to Your Heart     *24*

Making Peace with the Past     *34*

Balancing Work and Family     *41*

Seeing Yourself As You Are     *49*

Checking Your Progress and Setting Goals     *56*

The Perfect Day    *65*

Managing Motivation    *71*

Chill Out!    *81*

Listening to and Learning from Others    *88*

Scaling New Heights    *97*

If You Always Do What You've Always Done . . .    *104*

Are You Waiting Until You're Thin to Live?    *110*

Asking for Help    *116*

Where Can I Cash My Reality Check?    *123*

Getting Up with the Cows    *130*

Finding the Courage to Face Your Fears    *136*

You Can't Please Everyone . . .    *142*

Letting Go    *148*

Reaching Out to Others    *156*

Stay the Course    *162*

Put Your Body in Motion, Your Mind Will Follow    *168*

Seeds of Faith    *174*

Making Mistakes, Then Making Some More    *180*

Winning Your Angel Wings    *185*

Getting Focused and Staying Focused    *193*

Finding a Role Model—and Being One    *200*

Don't Be in a Hurry . . .    *207*

Counting Your Blessings    *214*

Finding the Heart to Begin    *221*

Handling Difficult People
and the Obstacle Course of Life    *229*

No More Being a Victim!    *240*

Resting on Your Laurels    *248*

Why Now Is the Best Time    *257*

If Your Best Is Good Enough for God,
Let It Be Good Enough for You    *265*

*String
of
Pearls*

# Introduction

---

*W*hen I first began sharing my Healthy Exchanges recipes, people weren't satisfied just learning how to cut their sugar and fat intake. They wanted real help in handling life's challenges—some that were food-related, and many that were not. Their requests encouraged me almost a decade ago to start writing a newsletter focused on "living healthy in the real world."

I decided that each monthly issue should provide not only dozens of new recipes but also a real boost of inspiration and practical advice by way of my editor's column. In just a few hundred words, which I now call "Straight From the Heart," I offer my thousands of subscribers my down-to-earth suggestions for ways to cope with the physical, psychological, and emotional issues they face every day.

When I created my HELP program and book a few years later, my readers welcomed it as a road map to the destination of healthy living for a lifetime; but even as its four parts—**H**ealthy eating, moderate **E**xercise, **L**ifestyle changes, **P**ositive attitude—provided a framework for that journey, hundreds of letters and phone calls asked for more guidance and direction.

This, then, is my answer—straight from the heart.

**String of Pearls** is a new kind of "recipe" book for me to write. This time, instead of outlining flavorful dishes that are quick and easy to prepare, I will share my recipes for living a happier, healthier, more complete life. Instead of stirring up pots of healthy ingredients, I want to stir *you* up, to get you thinking about how you are living your life, and why I believe you are capable of creating the life you want.

But what really sets me and my HELP program apart from all the other weight-loss programs out there in Slenderella land? How am I different from the other inspirational "gurus" who offer visions of a healthier you?

I believe it's my emphasis on Positive Attitude, which in turn leads to self-acceptance. Without that at the core of your life, your efforts to change are too often doomed to failure. When you fully understand that self-value comes from within, not from other people, you're free to become the person you most want to be.

I've always been a very practical, down-to-earth person, and the quality I value most is common sense. It's at the very heart of everything I share about healthy living. You see, I live in the Real World, and I know that most other people do, too. We can't exist on small portions of bland diet food or spend endless hours at the health club for the rest of our lives.

But we **can** learn to change our lives for the better.

We **can** learn to eat healthy food in moderation.

We **can** find the time for a fifteen-minute walk.

We **can** choose to set reasonable goals and map a way to reach them.

And we can only do this when we recognize our power to change, and move forward with a positive attitude.

I want to help you do just that. ***String of Pearls*** is the best way I know to offer the support you need.

My philosophy has always been that you can't "cram" anything down people's throats and expect it to change their lives. I never take the position that my way is the only way. Instead, I believe in offering suggestions, trying to get people to look at things differently. If they're not finding the solution to what is troubling them, maybe I can point the way.

I've thought long and hard about why size 10s turn to me for inspiration and tell me I'm their role model. Or why people young enough to be my children or old enough to be my parents ask me for help. I've spoken hundreds of times before all kinds of groups, including hospital staffs and health professionals far more educated than I am. And yet they have treated me as a kind of authority, and responded with positive energy to much of what I had to say. Why? Where does my authority come from? Why should anyone take my advice, or reshape their goals according to what I share with them? I'm convinced it's because they recognized that what I discussed and described came from life experience—from tackling life's problems head-on. By referring to my own history and responding to the problems of the many people who've visited with me in person, by phone, by mail, or by e-mail, I've been able to turn my empathy and my listening ear into practical, commonsense advice that can make a difference.

It's a little like listening to Grandma's view of the world—practical and spiritual all at once. I've come to believe that life is too short and too special to spend it constantly worrying, and through experience and prayer I've discovered that we are better off enjoying today because we never really know how many tomorrows we'll be granted. So it's important to find your best way of living physically, emotionally, and spiritually in order to fulfill your purpose on this earth.

***String of Pearls*** will share my thoughts, ideas, and techniques for building and sustaining self-esteem, using examples from my life and those of others who have shared their stories with me. I hope you will find in this little book a true companion, a friend to confide in, and a source of comfort in trying times.

## Why "String of Pearls"?

Why am I calling this little volume ***String of Pearls***?

Each of these chapters contains insights precious to me that I hope may point you down a path to greater happiness and fulfillment.

Each is polished by hard work, burnished by experience.

Each may seem meaningful alone, but when taken together, these chapters can help create a life of beauty, strength, and durability.

And the final product is more than the sum of its parts.

Where does the image of "string of pearls" come from? In part, it's that along the way I've discovered that the "secret of life" is no one big thing but lots of little things that add up to complete enjoyment. Joining these moments and revelations together, the big ones and the littler ones, is what brings us the most pleasure and satisfaction. (I also admit to being inspired by Glenn Miller's wonderful song called "String of Pearls," a joyful instrumental that echoes my emotions about this book!) I've always loved all kinds of jewelry, and what I especially like about pearls is that they're soft, not loud, not "in your face," adornment. They'll complement any woman's appearance, but as a supporting actor, not the prima donna.

***String of Pearls*** will provide, in written form, the experience of visiting with me one-on-one on the phone or in person. Because people have bared their souls to me, reaching out and asking for help instead of wallowing in self-pity, I want to give back to them a sense of self-worth, an appreciation of their value during a time of crisis, and a path to self-acceptance and self-realization. The goal of this book is not to help anyone lose weight. Instead, it is to help all people feel good about themselves.

I've always taken so much comfort in the Serenity Prayer used by many twelve-step recovery programs, but meaningful for all of us. It says, "God grant me the serenity to accept the things I cannot change, the courage to change the things I can, and the wisdom to know the difference."

I'm aiming to help my readers find all three, as I did: the serenity that I feel about the size-14 hips that will always be one size larger than the rest of me; the courage it took for a forty-six-year-old Iowa housewife to begin a speaking career when she'd never spoken before a group; and the wisdom I've earned over time by sifting through the experiences and emotions that I've confronted and shared with others.

People are so often tempted to resist their imperfections, more willing to experience frustration and failure in a search for ideal bodies or to live up to the expectations of others instead of channeling their desire for change toward possible miracles. I want to change that, to focus that energy and yearning on what's truly important—and what, like a string of pearls, will endure.

I often share the story of the rings on my fingers, one for each year I've sustained my original healthy living goals and weight loss. Each one is a visible reminder of how far I have come in finding and strengthening my own self-image, in discovering the work I believe God meant for me to do. When I sometimes face doubts or feel unfocused, I look to Him for the strength to go on—and to my hands for a vivid reminder of what I promised myself so long ago.

Just as each of those rings on my fingers recalls for me the experiences and accomplishments of each of the past ten years, so does this "string of pearls," this collection of life wisdom, bring back the memories of a lifetime for me, memories I want to share with you.

With this book, I invite you into what I call my "positive attitude room"—the place in my home I've chosen to celebrate my accomplishments, remember the inspirations that sustained me through challenges great and small, and strengthen my deep commitment to myself and to living the best life I can.

I want to be very clear that this is not a book to be read at one sitting. I hope this book will be a "work-your-work-book"—

a kind of lifestyle journal that encourages you, the reader, to take action. It's perfect for dipping into, flipping through, or reading a few pages before bed or first thing in the morning. This book lets you take home a piece of me, so when you need someone to listen or talk to, I'll be there.

I've subtitled this book "Recipes for Living Well in the Real World." I want you to walk with me out of the kitchen and begin creating a healthy life in the rest of the house, and in the world beyond. My stories and parables reflect my "velvet glove" approach to problem solving. The message comes through, but it's not preachy. I'd rather say, after listening to someone share his or her story, "Have you thought about this?" instead of "You must do this."

Just as financial whiz Suze Orman speaks to your relationship with money, so I want to help you tackle the emotional challenges of life—your relationships with others, your feelings about yourself and what the world has thrown your way. As the years pass, we know without doubt that our days on this earth are not infinite. We want to get the most possible enjoyment out of the days, weeks, months, and years we have left. But there are days when we can't help but feel that even if we have all the pieces to the puzzle that is our lives, we don't have them in the right places.

I hope *String of Pearls* will help guide you as you make your own journeys toward good health—emotional health, physical health, and of course spiritual health, too.

Try to think of me as a good friend, *not your mother,* and see this book not as something you'll read today and forget tomorrow. Leave it on the nightstand by your bed, so it will be there when you need it. I don't want to smother or overwhelm you with a million exercises, menus, or mantras. I hope together we can find a comfort zone of sharing our deepest feelings and concerns, and that together we can arrive at some new choices and goals that will shape a more satisfying future.

## Change Is Hard— and Making Excuses Is Easy

I like to say that all BIG accomplishments begin with *small* feats well done. Sometimes we do something so simple it seems wrong to call it an accomplishment, and so we downplay a small positive act. Or maybe it seems that no matter what we do, it's just not good enough.

That's why everything I do begins with **Positive Attitude.** As the Bible tells us, the last shall be first, and when it comes to HELP, the program I live by, the *P* for Positive Attitude is the most important thing—and the most elusive to capture.

**H**—Healthy recipes abound in all kinds of cookbooks.

**E**—Moderate exercise is available to almost anyone who is willing to put on a pair of walking shoes and head out the door.

**L**—Lifestyle changes are taught at weight-loss organizations, at hospital support groups, and at health clubs.

But **P**—Positive Attitude—has to come from deep within you. No one can teach you to cultivate it. No one can give it to you as a present. You can't buy it at any cost anywhere. And you for sure can't steal it. You have to earn it daily by doing small things right and feeling good about yourself as you do them.

Each new day gives you a fresh opportunity to do the best you can . . . *the best you can*, and then get on with life! **You don't expect more from yourself than you can give—and you don't settle for less.**

## *How I Earned My Own "String of Pearls"*

For years I struggled, wanting quick and easy answers, hoping for a miracle, wishing on stars, and being slowly and surely driven to depression by my inability to find a healthy way to live. I was at my wit's end when I finally saw the first glimmer of a light that January day almost ten years ago.

There was no going back, I decided at long last. I turned my health and weight dilemma over to God and prayed for the guidance to do what I had to do in His honor and glory to recapture my health.

I asked for the wisdom to accept myself with all my imperfections, and the strength to live a healthy lifestyle one day at a time. In that moment, with more than one hundred pounds to lose and more questions than answers, I finally experienced self-acceptance. I realized that I was a person of value no matter what size my hips were. After all, God created me with big hips. He just didn't put the extra padding on them! I had been taught that, with God, all things are possible, but accepting the full meaning of that teaching took me nearly forty-six years.

What did I want to accomplish, with God's help? For most of my life, I'd prayed to lose weight or to fit into a particular dress. And I wanted it without earning it. I wasn't asking for what I truly needed . . . until January 4, 1991, when my daily prayer was transformed. On that day, I asked with hope and humility, "Please, God, help me help myself just for today."

Intuitively, I knew that God expects more from me than just praying or repeating inspirational quotes. He expects me to do my part each day, to do the best I can . . . *the best I can*. That was the secret I'd been looking for all my life, and the answer I sensed would change everything I did from that moment on.

I truly believe:

**Prayers without Work are doomed to failure;**
**Work without Prayers won't be sustained long-term;**
**But Prayers combined with Work create Miracles**.

And I'm one. You can be, too.

If you've ever watched the movie *Pollyanna,* you know exactly what I mean by Positive Attitude. Pollyanna exuded Positive Attitude. She looked for the silver lining in every cloud—and she usually found it. *Pollyanna* is one of my favorite movies. I watched it again and again with my kids as they were growing up whenever it was featured on TV. My precious grandsons gave me a video of it for my birthday not long ago. It's been great to relive the emotion and excitement of the movie all over again with Zach and Josh.

Why is it such a special story? Because Pollyanna was able to change an entire town with her sunny disposition and her Positive Attitude. Just think what a daily dose of Positive Attitude could do for your life!

Positive Attitude changed me from a failed professional

dieter into a healthy and successful middle-aged grandmother, at peace with my size-14 hips.

I wear my own String of Pearls with pride. I think of those moments strung together, those experiences that have shaped and transformed my understanding of myself and my loved ones. Each time I remember one, I polish it with the soft cloth of clear-eyed reminiscence, seeing where it fits into the perfect circle that is life. And because so much of my recent life is a public one, I have benefited from hearing your stories too, sharing the powerful emotions, the ups and downs, that people have revealed to me, in their letters, their phone calls, and those precious times we've visited together after a bookstore appearance or a cooking class.

Recently, a woman came up to me in a Wal-Mart not far from my home in DeWitt, Iowa. I was shopping for my daughter when she appeared and said, "JoAnna? I've got to tell you something. You really changed my life. Remember when you spoke to the Army Corps of Engineers at Rock Island [Illinois]? You held up those size-28 pants and talked about being so overweight and having no energy. I sat there in my own size 28 pants, feeling so tired and depressed and stuck. But after listening to you, I decided that if you could do something about it, I could too. Now, a year and a half later, I'm wearing a size 10/12, and I walk every day." Her daughter stood next to her mother, and the tears in her eyes made my own well up with emotion. I did remember giving that talk, and recalled the moment when I pulled out those slacks for the thousandth time. I'd actually thought, just for a flash, "Oh, here I go again, telling the same old story of the slacks." This encounter made it clear, as nothing else could, that a story about changing my life, no matter how often I'd told it, still had the power to help others change theirs!

Some changes are harder to see than others, of course. Instead of being about weight loss or getting physically fit, maybe they involve giving up smoking or speaking up for yourself instead of remaining silent. But every time someone shares with me that I've contributed in some small way to a life change for her or him, I feel an amazing energy rush through my body. I'm refreshed by knowing that I helped, and it strengthens my own commitment to take good care of myself.

I'm just one stop on life's eventful journey for most people, though. They may pick up one of my books because they want to lose weight, and a blueprint for life changes begins to emerge. Maybe they say, well, I can't cook like this all the time, but maybe I'll use her recipes three nights a week. Or perhaps they will decide, I'll call up a friend and make a date to go walking tomorrow morning. By remodeling one thing about their lives, they may discover that everything looks different. One change can be a powerful catalyst for other changes. Someone says aloud, "Hmm, I did this; now maybe I could do something more." And sometimes, just sometimes, the trigger for that change is a visual one, like me holding up those stretched-out size-28 pants. I can never know who's already seen them, and who's looking at them with fresh eyes, ready to respond. There's a famous saying in Zen Buddhism, "When the student is ready, the teacher will come." But who those teachers are is a kind of mystery. It may not be your doctor who makes the strongest impression when you're feeling hopeless about ever controlling your blood sugar or building stronger bones. Sometimes it's a neighbor's diagnosis of diabetes or a hug from a grandson who asks, "Grandma, will you marry me when I grow up?" or a celebrity you listen to on late-night television. Something lights a fire inside you and gives you the impetus to make a change.

No one can know for sure when a revolutionary idea will penetrate your consciousness, or when it will be the right time for your heart and soul to accept an idea. I've received so many letters over the years from people who said, "I've seen you lots of times and I always found what you had to say interesting. But since I didn't need your recipes, I never took it a step further. But now I've been diagnosed with diabetes (or high cholesterol or a heart problem) and I'm so glad to know what to do."

There's a line from *Hamlet* that ends, "The readiness is all." Making even small changes requires a kind of readiness, just as making big ones does. Sometimes you are not ready to hear a particular truth or to accept guidance, but when you are, I hope you will be fortunate enough to find what you need at that moment.

I know that I wouldn't be doing what I'm doing if God hadn't put certain people in my path at the right time. So much would never have happened if not for a number of individuals; the unique way the events of my life have unfolded has brought me to the point I'm at now. Not all of what I've learned along the way has been good, but it's all taught me something that's helped me grow as a person. (And truly, we might not appreciate what is good, if not for the bad things that provide a vivid contrast. I've had occasion to remind myself of this from time to time, prodding my stubborn self and saying that I had to go through what I went through to reach the here and now.)

That's Positive Attitude for you!

Now, not every pearl is a keeper. You need to sift through the moments of your life and choose what to cherish. Only Adam and Eve were given the Garden of Eden; the rest of us have to deal with an imperfect world. But I don't long for perfection; I wouldn't know how to live there. Instead, I struggle every day to find the positive in the life I've got.

I've called my work both a mission and a ministry, and sometimes people have wondered why I saw it just that way. To me, a mission is a life purpose, a spiritual journey, and a ministry the opportunity to reach out to others. I've been blessed to find both, sharing and teaching what I've been blessed to learn.

Most of us have heard of ministers who thunder and threaten, who insist there is only one way, whose favorite three words are Thou Shalt Not . . . , and whose sermons are the kind you can't wait to escape.

Well, that's not what you're going to find in here. I want my mini-sermons, my meditations and revelations, to be so enjoyable that you'll continue to seek them out over weeks and months and even years. My message is one of hope, along with the knowledge of how to address some of life's toughest problems. I believe that God gives us talents on this earth, and that we're meant to use them for the betterment of others. With this book, I'm so happy to share with you the pearls of life wisdom I've polished over the years.

May your life always be as precious and luminous as a beautiful string of pearls.

*Jo Anna*

# Learning to Accept What You Cannot Change

*First ask yourself: What is the worst that can happen? Then prepare to accept it. Then proceed to improve on the worst.*

—DALE CARNEGIE

𝒥'm married to a younger man. He was younger when I met him. He was younger when I married him. And he's *still* younger than I am.

I married Cliff because I love him. I didn't let the fact that I'm older than he is by a few years keep us apart. I recognized that it was a fact of life I couldn't change, and I learned to accept it.

(Actually, it could turn out to be very smart to marry a younger man, since women tend to live longer than men do. This way, we'll be together the rest of our lives, if we're lucky!)

You may wonder why I mention something that seems so minor when I talk about accepting what you cannot change. But have you ever known a woman who had very specific ideas about the kind of man she would want to marry, or even date? Maybe he'd have to look a certain way, or have a certain type of job. For many women, a prospective romantic partner has to be a few years older. Why? Perhaps so she'll always feel younger when they're together. Or maybe she worries that in marrying a younger man, she'd be considered a "cradle robber" or foolish.

I wasn't a young girl when I met Cliff, and I'd already learned that what really mattered to me had nothing to do with age. I also knew that his age was a fact about him I could never change. I accepted it, we got married, raised some great kids, built a business together, and continue to be very happy. (We celebrated our twentieth anniversary just as the century was coming to a close in 1999!)

For me, the fact of marrying a younger man was an easy thing to accept. Not everything about my life has been quite that simple, especially when it came to my body, my weight, and my sense of self.

For years, I thought that if I deprived myself, criticized my body, exercised harder, and ate almost nothing, I could get rid of my hips, which have always been a size larger than the rest of me. Well, I did all those things, and all I succeeded in doing was damaging my health and crushing my self-esteem. Eventually, I learned to follow a healthy lifestyle and lost the extra weight, but even when I became a happy and healthy size 12, my hips were still hanging on at size 14.

Did I lock myself in the house and refuse to go out? Did I sign up for liposuction or wrap layers of Saran Wrap around my body in hopes of sweating off those curves? Did I decide, "Now it's time for a crash diet or a liquid diet or a juice fast?"

I did not.

I said to myself, "JoAnna, God made you and He made you hippy. You've done your part and done your best, but some things aren't going to change. Now, you can accept it and get on with your life, or you can wallow in unhappiness the rest of your days." Okay, I admit it, I get a little melodramatic when I talk to myself sometimes. But this was an important realization for me. After all, I'd lived with my hips for years, and accepting that I'd always be hippy was a big attitude change.

It was also amazingly liberating. For the first time in years, maybe ever, I could look at myself in the mirror without frowning. I could try on a new outfit and say, "This looks good on me." Not, "This would look good on me if it weren't for my hips sticking out there!"

That's not to say that I don't try to use a few fashion tricks to diminish my lack of "perfect" proportions. I do all I can to emphasize my best features with the clothes and colors I choose and the jewelry I accessorize with.

Does all this sound like a contradiction of what I said earlier? It's not, not really. I believe, just as the song says, in "ac-cen-tu-ating" the positive aspects of my appearance. But at the same time, I accept myself—hips and all.

Remember the classic Serenity Prayer I mentioned in the Introduction? We ask God for serenity to accept the things we cannot change, the courage to change the things we can, and the wisdom to know the difference. In those plain words, we're inviting the help and guidance of a Higher Power in dividing what we have to handle in life into two categories: what we CAN change and what we CANNOT. Once we've made the necessary distinctions, we're ready to take action—where action can be taken.

But because action takes effort and guts, we also ask for courage in making the changes that are in our power. Knowing what to do isn't enough. Recognizing what it will take to change what we can is only the first step. After that, it's time for the real work to begin.

But taking action is only part of the Serenity Prayer, and too often it's the part that we give the most attention to. We focus on how we can change, and why we must change, and how our lives will unfold once we commit ourselves to becoming changed human beings. Certainly, when the goal is to stop unhealthy or dangerous habits such as abusing alcohol or prescription drugs, changing behavior is the most visible focus of the pursuit of that end.

But acceptance is just as important as making changes. In some ways, it's even more significant, and it requires as much or more "wisdom" to make peace with what *is*. Too often, even when we succeed in making behavioral changes, our unwillingness to reach a point of self-acceptance can sabotage our efforts and even bring the hard-fought transformation to a grinding halt!

Why does this happen? Why does making peace with what you can't do anything about cause us even more grief than what we have to struggle to change?

I suspect it's because we don't want to acknowledge that some things in our lives are beyond our control, that no matter how much we may want something to be true, it's not going to happen. Facing that reality can hurt. Coming to terms with that fact can be depressing. But if we surrender to negativity on this point, we're dooming our efforts to change for good. Even worse, we're denying ourselves an important opportunity to heal pain that we may have buried for years.

I've known a great many women who were diagnosed with breast cancer, and while each one handled her diagnosis and treatment in her own way, I noticed that many of the women who were more accepting of the fact of the disease seemed better able to face what came next. I've discussed this observation with medical professionals who work with cancer patients, and they told me that I was on the mark. By accepting where you are at the moment, you can focus your considerable energies on where you want to go next. Cancer cells can't be argued with or persuaded to disappear by refusing to acknowledge their existence. But they can be fought in a variety of different ways.

Perhaps that's an extreme example, but the principle makes sense to me. Here's another: Suppose your daughter absolutely loves basketball, but at five-foot-one, she's a real long shot to make her high school team. She hasn't grown an inch in years, so she's probably stuck with her height. But she's not without options. She can practice foul shooting until she's practically perfect, and work at guarding much taller girls until she convinces the coach what an asset she'll be to the team (both the WNBA and the NBA have hired some very short but brilliant players). If she doesn't want to give up her dream of being part of the team, she can volunteer to help manage it or work behind the scenes in some other way. She can try to organize an after-school league for all the girls who love the sport but don't qualify for the varsity squad. She can decide to pursue a sport where being tall is less of an issue (soccer? gymnastics? track?).

She can do just about anything except stretch herself on a rack until she's half a foot taller! What's important is that she recognize that she's not stuck. In fact, sometimes these kinds of obstacles are the inspiration for greatness, the spark that ignites a dream that hadn't existed before someone ran into a brick wall or someone who said, "No, you can't."

But often the first impulse is to say it yourself, even before someone else does. I've gotten hundreds of letters and e-mails from people who feel defeated by circumstances, and I've spoken with many women and men who can't quite see beyond the obstacles they perceive.

In many cases, the obstacle is very real: coping with a disease like lupus or a physical infirmity like arthritis of the knee requires special effort, but it can be done. And making an effort to lose weight and get healthy even when you're smack in the middle of menopause isn't impossible. It just may take more time, more patience, and more determination than you've previously been willing to devote to the task.

Most of those who hear me tell my own story tend to focus on the accomplishment of losing 130 pounds and keeping them off for nearly a decade. But my weight-loss success is only part of the story. When I reached my lowest point physically and emotionally back in 1991, I was dangerously overweight, but I also had problems with high blood pressure, arthritis, gout, and cholesterol. Not only that, but my arthritic feet sometimes hurt so much when I got out of bed that I couldn't walk on the soles of my feet for at least ten to fifteen minutes. I could easily have convinced myself that exercise, any exercise, could not be part of my lifestyle because everything HURT. But I checked with my doctor, who encouraged me to do whatever I could, until it began to feel better. Well, one place I felt better was in the pool, so that's where I started walking, back and forth, back and forth, until the pounds started coming off. And when spring arrived, I made sure I had an especially well padded seat on my bike so I'd be comfortable when I rode around DeWitt, not setting any speed records but burning calories just the same.

Not long ago, I received a letter from a woman who explained that she'd been cooking with my healthy recipes, but she wasn't exercising at all. She left for work when it was still dark out, so she didn't feel safe walking in her neighborhood, and never had time in the evenings because she cared for an aging parent. She couldn't afford to join a gym at the present moment, she added, and while she occasionally worked out to a video, she knew it wasn't enough. Did I have any other ideas, she asked?

I did. (You're not surprised, are you?)

I used to ride my bike the two miles between my house and the office building, which gave me a great opportunity to decompress from the tensions of the workday and also to get those muscles moving. But now my office is in my house, and the building that houses the print shop and our small staff is only a few minutes' walk away.

I also don't get up to the Hart Center, our community health club, very often anymore, to use the pool or walk indoors with friends. It's a much longer drive, and besides that, my best time for getting exercise in tends to be very early in the morning. But here in Iowa it's cold and dark in those hours, and I don't like the idea of bundling up like the Michelin man to walk up and down our country roads at 5 A.M.

It's quite a little list of obstacles, isn't it? I could easily say, "Oh well, no time or place to exercise, so I'll just let it slide until spring is here." But I won't do that. Feeling good in my body and about my body is just too important to me. So I've come up with an alternative that works for me, even if some of my friends chuckle at my "method."

I walk my house.

I wrote about this technique in my HELP book, but it's an entirely different experience now from doing laps around our little cottage that was home for most of Cliff's and my married life until now. The new house has more room to cover, more stairs to climb, and more nooks and crannies to weave in and out of. I wore a pedometer once to figure out how much ground I cover as I move from room to room briskly, getting my heart pumping while the rest of the world is still asleep. What's nice about walking indoors? No rocks to trip over, no barking dogs running after you, no cars to avoid, no layers of winter clothing to zip up and pull on so I don't freeze!

I mention this personal example because it makes the point again: I can't make the sun come up earlier; I can't make the Iowa winters less bleak and dreary; I can't move our house back to town. But I also can't give up on myself, and so I've accepted what I can't change about my exercise time—and I've figured out a way to make it work.

There are wonderful chair exercise tapes for people who can't stand and work out; there are twenty-four-hour gyms in some cities for people who work the night shift; there are more kinds of exercise videos than I ever imagined, so anyone can find one that is "just right." And as for making my peace with menopause, I can tell you it wasn't easy, but since I couldn't stop the wheels of time from turning, I had to find a way to live with the changes in my body. Some things I tried didn't work, but I kept reading and asking questions and—oh, yes—promising myself that the worst of it would eventually pass. And you know what—it did!

### A Pearl to Polish

*Accepting what you can't change saves a great deal of energy—energy that you can channel into making your life as happy and full as possible. And "wising up" to what you can change will help you focus some of that energy on doing just that. Today, choose three things about your life or yourself that you can't change, and say aloud, "I accept* ~~the things that~~ *I know it's something that will always be true, and I can live with that." Then, list three things about yourself or your life that you know you can change, and say aloud one way you will tackle each of them. Then make a start, today. Tomorrow, or in the next few days, add another tactic or two to your list. Baby steps first, then bigger ones, but as Henry David Thoreau said, "Keep moving in the direction of your dreams."*

*[handwritten annotations:]*

I can't change right now. Time, paying a babysiter.

I can chang my weight My Eating My Commitment to Do an Exercise that works for me. Exp. walking.

My Eating — I can change it By eating more greens.

My Weight — Pick a time to go for a walk Even w/ Callie.

My Commitment — Do small (start slow) 10-15min work outs 2-3 times a week.

Start Tomorrow 5-12-14 Eat well/Greens go for a walk do a short workout

# Listening to Your Heart

---

*Champions aren't made in gyms. Champions are made from something they have deep inside them—a desire, a dream, a vision. They have to have the skill, and the will. But the will must be stronger than the skill.*

—MUHAMMAD ALI

*E*very month in my newsletter I answer reader questions about all kinds of topics, and regularly I am asked about how to handle situations involving food. Not long ago I received an e-mail that asked for help handling an upcoming Valentine's Day. "I just know I'll eat more than my share of my child's candy hearts," she wrote. "How do I stop myself before I start?"

I didn't have to think for more than a moment before starting to draft my reply. The answer is a simple one, but knowing the right answer isn't enough. You have to *want* to stop yourself before you start, I began, or you probably won't stop yourself. And you have to want to stop yourself in both your head and in your heart. If both don't agree to stop at the same time, then your body will be fighting a kind of Civil War and more than likely, the candy hearts will come out the victor!

It helps to examine the situation you're faced with: Will you be buying the candy hearts or will someone else be giving them to your kids? If you are buying them, then the easiest solution is to buy very small boxes (one for each child) and distribute them. Crisis solved. But if others are providing these tasty treats to your children, and you've received more than they can (or should) eat, why not suggest donating the excess to a local food bank so less fortunate children can enjoy a Valentine's Day treat, too?

The bottom line is, you need to pause for a moment before putting candy hearts or anything else in your mouth, then ask yourself two questions: first, Do you really want to eat this now? and second, Will you be accountable to yourself for it if you do? If you truly want it, and you plan for it, enjoy it—and move on. But more often than not, I suspect you will decide to pass. After a moment's reflection, you may see the choice more clearly and know that your nibbling of candy hearts on Valentine's Day in the past was more an unconscious eating activity. There they were in the bowl on the table: your hand reached out, took a bunch, tossed them into your mouth—and crunch, crunch, crunch, you'd chewed and swallowed a few hundred calories of sugar that left you feeling guilty and out of control.

Now consider another scenario: It's Valentine's Day, and you've always loved candy hearts—for their sweetness, for the little humorous sayings like "Be Mine," and for how they reminded you of happy times in childhood. You decided that a box of candy hearts would be a perfect afternoon snack, and you planned for it, made a note of the calories, and actually sat down to enjoy your chosen sweets. You ate them one at a time, unlike in past years, when you gobbled down at least six or eight in a mouthful. When the box was empty, you smiled, wished yourself a happy Valentine's Day, and went back to work or off to do your errands. You felt good, not guilty.

Now wouldn't that be a great way to handle the situation? And you can do it.

Every healthy eating choice begins in your mind, not your mouth. That's why you've got the tools and power you need to cope with any eating challenge, any special occasion. You just have to be willing to use them to your advantage!

How? By getting in touch with the positive, optimistic, hopeful, and strong part of yourself that may be buried deep under mountains of frustration, layers of anger, piles of bitterness, and stacks of shame. Those negative "weights" may be weighing you down and holding you back from moving in the direction of your dreams.

Some people who insist they are eager, even desperate, to lose weight or improve their health follow up those comments by listing all the reasons they just can't do it—or can't do it right now:

- They've always hated vegetables, and fruit doesn't satisfy them in any way, shape, or form, except perhaps in pie.
- They grew up eating Mom's fried chicken and can't face eating poultry any other way.
- They find walking boring, think working out to exercise videos at home feels silly, but feel too embarrassed to join a gym.

- They have no time for support group meetings, or they're too shy to join, or they think there's no reason to pay when they already know how to lose weight.
- They're terrible at writing things down, so they can't keep a food journal.
- They're awful cooks, so there's no question of trying to prepare healthy recipes.
- They love to eat so much, they could never be satisfied dining on moderate portions.
- They feel like crying when everyone else at the restaurant is munching on buttered rolls and they've ordered salad with a light dressing.
- They're convinced it's too much trouble to plan meals in advance, or they prefer to be spontaneous and eat whatever is handy.
- They have already decided that the most fattening foods taste the best, and so they can't stick to an eating plan that eliminates creamy sauces and oily dressings.
- They're tired of being left out of the fun when everyone else is drinking and nibbling during happy hour.
- They're on a tight budget, and healthy foods like fresh vegetables, ready-made salads, or the leanest meats are too costly. (Though they still manage to slip bags of chips and boxes of cookies into the shopping cart, because they're on sale!)

Do you see yourself in any of these comments? Have you been blocking your own way because you're in a mental rut that says, "Change is too hard"? Is it possible that by viewing your behavior through clearer eyes, you might figure out how to counter each of these obstacles—and achieve what you say is your heart's dearest desire?

Let's try it together.

If you've never been a fan of eating raw fruits and vegetables, or you feel they give you gas, then what could you do to cope? You could bake the best-looking apples you can find, pouring some light maple syrup over them before sliding them into the oven. You could stir some tasty canned fruit in its own juice into your favorite flavors of sugar-free gelatin. You could try some new recipes, including my own Healthy Exchanges ones, that incorporate canned veggies like corn, beans, and carrots into tasty casseroles. You could reward yourself for munching celery and carrot sticks by stirring up a terrific dip using fat-free sour cream, which tastes almost as decadent as the real thing. You could even try one of those products that promises to help your body cope with high-fiber foods, like Beano. The important point is, you've got options.

Next up, your childhood comfort food, fried chicken. I'd never try to tell you that your only choices are the deep-fried kind or boiled boneless breasts that lack flavor or eye appeal, but you'd be surprised how many people think that it's true. There are literally hundreds (if not thousands) of ways to cook chicken and turkey that don't require a deep fryer or a gallon of oil, but you do need an open mind and a willingness to sample different approaches. There are terrific baked "fried" chicken recipes that will surprise anyone who tries them, as well as many other ways of preparing poultry that are both good and good for you. Don't accept defeat when it comes to substitutions—keep trying until you find what pleases you and your family!

If you agree with the people who find walking dull or videos silly, you may be letting your own dissatisfaction with yourself get the best of you. Yes, walking is a repetitive motion, but because it doesn't require the intense concentration of, oh, kickboxing, you can allow your mind and eyes to wander. In the course of an hour's walk outside, you could feast your senses on everything you see around you; in the space of a half hour on the treadmill, you could watch your favorite sitcom from childhood in reruns and relive those carefree days. If the videos you've tried make you feel awkward or out of step, they're just the wrong ones for you. But somewhere out there are tapes and teachers who will capture your attention and lead you to better health— you've just got to keep looking for them. If you love dancing but hate exercise, there are line dancing and salsa tapes. And if you're too uncomfortable with your body to lift weights at the gym, buy a pair of dumbbells and a video that will teach you at home.

I get letters every day from people who use my recipes and attend weight-loss support group meetings, so I know how much help they can be for people with weight and health concerns. If you feel you're too busy to attend, why not make a list of the activities you do each week, and ask yourself which of them is less important to you right now than recapturing your health. Could you cut back on your volunteering one afternoon to make a meeting, or could your spouse take the car pool one evening so you'd be free to attend? Can you organize a support group at the office one lunchtime each week? Give yourself every opportunity to benefit from this valuable support, if it's right for you. Fear you're too shy to speak up, so you doubt you'd benefit from a group situation? I think you might surprise yourself once you start going and get comfortable in an environment that is welcoming and nonjudgmental. But even if you just listen, you're likely to get something out of it. And as for paying for a support group when you already "know" how to lose weight—let me just say this: Even when we know what to do, we don't always do it. For many people, a well-led group provides inspiration, fresh ideas, helpful techniques for coping with eating challenges, and much more. With the cost of health care ever rising, the price of attending a regular support meeting could be the best money you ever spent!

I'm not sure why you might resist the notion of writing down what you eat—maybe because it feels too much like homework? But seeing your choices in black and white can be a helpful tool on your journey to better health. It's partly about taking responsibility for what goes into your mouth; it's also good for learning to be honest with yourself, often after years of secretive eating. A food journal can help you recognize that you're eating the same things all the time, which could explain why you're experiencing a weight-loss plateau. And it can also provide encouragement that you're doing the right thing, and the scale is sure to show it—if not this week, then soon. So if keeping a food journal at least for the first few weeks or months of your new healthy lifestyle is standing between you and your heart's desire, why not promise yourself a little nonfood reward for each week that you write down your meals three to four days out of seven? An extra ten minutes on the phone with your daughter, perhaps, or a new shade of lipstick that you don't need but would enjoy trying.

For the bad cooks and the noncooks among you, I'm happy to have provided some of the easiest, most foolproof recipes on record! So even if you're convinced that boiling water is beyond you, or that milk curdles when you walk by, don't allow your history of failure in the kitchen to prevent you from getting healthy once and for all! My own sister Jeannie has always insisted she's a true noncook, and she manages to make terrific meals from my super-easy suggestions. Pick the fastest, pick the simplest, pick the foods you love so much you're willing to risk making a mess. Then just tune the radio to a feel-good station, read the recipe carefully, stir it up, set the timer, and prepare for some surprised but delighted applause from the family.

For those who can't be satisfied by moderate portions, or who feel so deprived because they're denying themselves a buttered roll, let me say this: Don't give up without trying to solve what feels like a problem. If it takes bigger portions to satisfy your appetite, emphasize high-volume foods prepared in lowfat ways. I know how it feels to want a hearty serving, so many of my recipe servings are a quarter of an eight-by-eight-inch pan. That's a big mound of food, believe me, and Cliff, my truck-drivin' man, digs in with a smile on his face when I serve my latest kitchen creation. Will you ever learn to be satisfied with less? Over time, as you begin to eat healthier and without deprivation, yes, especially because you know that after your tasty dinner tonight, there will be a good breakfast tomorrow, followed by a satisfying lunch, and another delicious dinner tomorrow night— with dessert! When it's no longer feast or famine at your table, "enough" isn't always as much as it used to be.

Have I got an answer for everything? Just about, since I've been answering reader questions in the newsletter for years, and taking questions at speaking engagements for a decade now! Obviously, different people require different answers, so not all these problems will be yours. But I hope that a few of these points hit home with you, and that my proposed solutions give you new hope of conquering a few more "mountains."

Whether it's planning meals in advance, or allotting more of your grocery budget to the foods that will get you and keep you healthy, you already know how to tackle the obstacles that appear to stand in your way. Most of the time, all that is required is a willingness to accept what is truly in your heart. Yes, you may long for those days of wine and roses, when you could drink a bottle of wine or a pitcher of margaritas and never suffer any health consequences from going a little overboard occasionally. But if your heart's goal is better health, you have to decide to do what you can to satisfy it. Sometimes, that means settling for a light beer or two, then switching to club soda while you're watching the Super Bowl or the People's Choice Awards. Sometimes, that means deciding to be a little less spontaneous when it comes to what you have for lunch each day at the office, maybe bringing a thermos of healthy soup to enjoy along with your turkey sandwich instead of gulping down three slices of pizza with extra cheese and pepperoni. Sometimes, that means stopping after just a spoonful or two of a favorite food that's very high in fat or sugar. You could focus on feeling deprived and deny yourself the pleasure of the taste, or you could listen to your heart, the voice inside your soul that says, "I'd rather feel healthy and look good than eat seconds of everything at the buffet." Some days, the voice may not speak loudly enough to persuade you to put down your fork, but the more you listen to what you truly want, the louder and stronger the voice soon becomes.

## *A Pearl to Polish*

*Only by listening to your heart can you deal with what stands in your way of achieving happiness. But before your heart can communicate what you most deeply want and need, you have to be ready to hear what it has to say. The next time you catch yourself making excuses for why you can't take a step toward better health, stop—and think about what it would take for you to retract that statement and rephrase it so you give yourself the chance to succeed. Focus on your want power, and you will find a way.*

I feel FAT/Inchada, Ugly, No wants of dressing nice cause I Feel ugly, I have no power to look better because I Feel & look fat.

I WANT TO LOOSE 12Lbs - I WANT TO Look &Feel Healthy & Sexy & Pretty. I need to Live Long to take Care of my Callie.

I want to be me again...... What an I going To Do to Get There.

1) Food Jurnal
2) Eat more Greens
3) Start Walking
4) keep Doing Kettle Bels 3Times week.
5) Reward My Self.

# Making Peace with the Past

*Close the door on the past. You don't try to forget the mistakes, but you don't dwell on it. You don't let it have any of your energy, or any of your time, or any of your space.*

—JOHNNY CASH

*M*ost people who've struggled with being overweight can provide extensive diaries of their temporary successes and devastating failures, even if they've never written down a word. The memories are specific and intense, refusing to fade away as so many other facts and faces from our pasts tend to do.

Of course, the pictures help us remember—in greater detail than we would like. When you're sitting with the family during a holiday meal, and someone pulls out a scrapbook or photo album, it's hard not to study these images of the past without thinking something like "Oh, yes, I'd just lost ten pounds on a juice fast, so I could fit into that purple dress. I never wore it again." Or, "How

I hate that picture of my brother's thirtieth birthday dinner! My face looks like a big round moon and my body is even worse." Or perhaps, "I remember thinking I was so fat when I was in college, but I would give anything to fit into that size 12 pantsuit now."

It's difficult to escape the past in pictures, unless you were "clever" enough to avoid being photographed. Do you have hundreds of photographs from your most memorable vacations, and you're not in any of them? Are you always carefully positioned behind everyone else so only your face can be seen in the picture? Have you ever torn up a photograph sent to you by a friend because you so detested how you looked in it?

If you answered "yes" to any of these questions, then you know exactly what I mean when I say that you have a history of failure to deal with. You've got photographic evidence of your inability to keep off the weight you lost on any of a dozen diets. You've got a nearly photographic memory of every miserable emotion you felt when you were part of a bridal party and couldn't fit into the dress, or when you had to shop in the maternity department, or when you weren't fit enough to get better than a D on the President's Physical Fitness Tests back in the sixties.

Good memories are precious and warm us, if we're lucky, all our lives long. But bad memories can have an even more powerful stranglehold on our hearts. They weigh us down emotionally, they stand in our way when we're contemplating life changes, and they can even be passed down to our children and grandchildren if we're not careful. That's no kind of legacy to share with the people you love, is it?

If you can identify with the notion of a history of failure, welcome to the club. We've got millions of members—but if we work together on this, I hope we can find a way to put that part of our history behind us, maybe silence it altogether.

First, we have to face the enemy and give it a name. Grab a pad of paper and begin by writing down the first ten things that come to mind under the heading: "I Have a History of Failure." Yes, you may feel some very painful twinges as you even scribble that line down, but they will soon pass. On your list, write down ten (just ten, that's plenty) recollections you have about failing to do what you wanted to do: the time you flunked your driver's license test (for the second time!), the experience of losing a job you enjoyed to downsizing, the pain of gaining back a lot of weight you lost for a special family occasion, the heartbreak of accepting that a marriage had ended. Can't think of ten? Well, you're a very lucky person! Most people who've survived a certain number of years on this earth have a history of failure that provides plenty of material for this exercise; life just isn't easy, no matter how hard you work at it, and setbacks and disappointments are part of it.

Okay, you've got your list? Now take a deep breath and study it for just a minute or two. Yup, I remember how terrible that one felt. Uh-huh, I cried for a week after that happened. Wallow for just this short interval of time in how failure makes you feel—hopeless? exhausted? depressed?

I'm certain you're feeling all of the above and more. Now don't despair, I'm getting to the point of all this "excavation" of the darker moments in your past.

Okay, it's time to take another sheet of paper and write at the top: "I Have a History of Success." Don't those words just give you a little burst of energy and hope? Now, take a few min-

*I Have A History of Success:*
*School*
*BS*
*MBA*
*Callie*
*Family*
*Health*
*Travel*
*Real State*
*Creative*
*GoGetter*
*Achiever*
*My 1st. Car*
*Book*

utes to write down as many big and little successes you can think of in your life. Give yourself credit for everything that made you feel like a winner, from acing a pop quiz in a difficult class to getting your college degree in your forties, from raising three basically healthy, happy kids to adulthood (definitely one of mine!) to giving a speech that terrified you. This list includes the church bazaar you organized, the house you redecorated on a shoestring, the flat tire you learned how to change all by yourself. And yes, include any times when you set a goal and reached it, even if that goal wasn't a lasting one. Losing weight counts; showing up at the gym three times a week for a month counts; passing your real estate broker's licensing test really counts!

Take about five to ten minutes (or longer if ideas keep pouring out of you). Use two or three sheets of paper if necessary. Write on the back if you run out of room. Keep going and going and going, just like that old Energizer bunny, until you have to stop and rest.

How do you feel now? Is the misery and sadness that filled you after the first list pushed to the very back of your brain? Or at least shoved way aside? Good. Focus on how reading your list of accomplishments feels, the little fires that begin to burn inside you, the glow of satisfaction fanned into a bonfire of intense pleasure.

Quite a difference, isn't there? Kind of like saying "I can" instead of "I can't," right?

Anyone who's read my books or newsletters knows how much I like to use little mottoes or slogans that crystallize what I'm trying to say. Sometimes they whisper their way into my consciousness while I'm working; sometimes they're shared with me by readers or colleagues. And when they're really good ones, I like to pass them on. So attention please, here's my success slogan for the day:

What's Past Is Past. **P**ositive **A**ttitude **S**tarts **T**oday.

Does that mean that I want you to pretend that your past experiences of failure don't exist? Not at all. But I do want you to benefit from acknowledging the power of positive attitude when it comes to coping with your past.

The past is part of who we are, what we feel, where we've been. But it's not the entire story. No matter what kind of past we've had up to this point, we don't have to live there anymore. We're not chained to what didn't work before, and we're not stuck in the mindset that made us feel helpless and hopeless. Instead, when we catch ourselves feeling less than confident because of past failures, we have a little phrase to pull out of our bag of tricks: What's Past Is Past. Positive Attitude Starts Today.

I'm on a roll now, I think. Here's another play on words that emphasizes moving ahead, not hanging back: **P**ick **A**nother **S**trategy **T**oday. If what you've done in the past hasn't gotten you what you want, Pick Another Strategy—and do it *Today!*

That's exactly what I look for in the Success Stories I choose for each issue of my monthly newsletter. What did you do, I ask the people whose stories I share, and what did you do that was different from what you'd been doing? What kept you going when boredom set in, and what kept you focused in busy, stressful times? To a man and to a woman, they turned their eyes and hearts to the future instead of wallowing in the past. In some cases, they had faced tragedy, and in others, terrifying health crises. For many, eating healthy was something positive that they could do after chemotherapy, or during grief counseling for the loss of a child. For some, whose roles as caretakers to aging parents, ill spouses, or disabled children were overwhelming, arranging to spend an hour at the gym two or three times a week made the difference between sustaining their sanity (and their own health!) and being weighed down with the responsibility of caring for loved ones.

One of my favorite letters came from a woman whose husband was recovering from a stroke. His speech had been affected, and for two years he hadn't said a word about the food he was served. One night, his wife prepared a peanut butter pie recipe of mine, and after his first bite, her husband said, "Good." It made her day when it happened, and it made my day when I read her note. Sometimes peanut butter has the power to heal what's ailing us, and what a comfort to find that we can still enjoy it in MODERATION while pursuing a healthy lifestyle!

No matter what has gone before—

No matter how many times you've regained weight you'd lost—

No matter how many disappointments you've experienced over the years when it came to getting into better shape—

No matter how frustrated you feel about the limitations your doctor has placed on you—

No matter how often you've tried to change your behavior and failed—

You don't have to stay mired in the past.

You don't have to live forever with the consequences of what you've done in the past.

You don't have to feel helpless in the face of a history of failure.

Because—

You have a history of success that outweighs your record of failure.

You're finally ready to say, "What's past is past."

You've got a new approach to an old problem because Positive Attitude Starts Today.

You've got a whole world of options whereas before you seemed to have none.

Now, why not Pick Another Strategy Today—and ease on down the road to a brighter future!

### *A Pearl to Polish*

*Every time you find a negative thought creeping into your brain, stop what you're doing at that moment (if you can) and actually say aloud, "STOP." Then, imagine a red light changing to green, and put your "foot on the gas." Accelerate forward with as much positive energy as you can churn up inside, and put the past behind you for keeps.*

# Balancing Work and Family

---

*Be aware of wonder. Live a balanced life—learn some and think some and draw and paint and sing and dance and play and work every day some.*

—ROBERT FULGHUM

For many years my favorite word has been *moderation,* but even as I was saying it, I wasn't always practicing it. Oh, I certainly followed the principle in my healthy lifestyle choices, where food and exercise were concerned. But when it came to setting goals and following my dreams, I discovered firsthand how passion and commitment could lead me down the path of exhaustion and overcommitment. I knew that moderation in all things was best, but I was so determined to share my message and grow my business that I got a little off track. Or truer yet, I found myself with a life completely out of balance.

When I say the word *balance,* what image do you get? Can

you see an ice skater or ballerina twirling on one magical point, somehow defying gravity and staying on her feet? Can you visualize a weight lifter straining to raise a heavy barbell overhead, hoping and praying that he won't be pulled to one side or the other by the weight? Or maybe you envision two kids playing on a seesaw, and riding up and down at a frantic pace, never finding that magical moment when both floated in the air, feet off the ground, perfectly even and still?

Well, I've discovered in the past couple of years that life is not *The Ed Sullivan Show*. You don't get extra credit by keeping more plates or balls in the air than all the other jugglers. Instead, most likely, your heart rate skyrockets, you feel a headache coming on, and you just know that sooner or later, you'll be picking up broken china off the floor!

I've always been a busy person, active, involved, even driven at times, and I think I was probably so busy I wasn't aware of what my over-full schedule was doing to me. Oh, I had moments of uneasiness and fatigue, but I figured they were due to not getting enough sleep the night before. Then I started to count the cost: I'd lost the time I always treasured for gardening; I didn't have the time I wanted with my grandkids, who were more wonderful to be with all the time; and I hadn't had time for activities I love, like sewing, for longer than I could remember.

Years ago, *Ms.* magazine used to call it the "click": a clear moment in time when you knew something had to change, when you finally recognized that the way things were wasn't right for you anymore. I heard the click loud and clear all of a sudden. I was leaving the house before 7 A.M. and not getting home until after 9 P.M. I was working nights and weekends, and often I would wake up at dawn to get in a few hours of writing before going in to the office. I was functioning on the outside, holding the fort and staying my usual calm. But there was an undercurrent I'd never really felt before, and I didn't know what it was.

That spring I was full of plans, new projects that would add to the workload but which I found very exciting to contemplate. Cliff and I had discussed opening Grandma Jo's Country Inn, a local B&B, and we'd gone so far as to have drawings made and even spoken to our contractor. A company was interested in marketing my frozen pies, and customers were even lined up and ready to go. Then three things happened in succession that brought the situation to a head:

First, my father-in-law had a stroke. Suddenly, though I felt good about the business, I began to think about how much longer Cliff's parents would be part of our lives.

Second, a good friend of ours lost his wife to cancer at quite a young age. Certain deaths hit you hard, and this was one of them. When I realized that this woman, who was younger than I was, would never see her daughter grow up, I felt absolutely shaken. I had two grandchildren already, and three on the way, and if I kept on the way I was, I would barely get to know them.

But it was the third troubling event, a truly defining, turn-around moment, that helped me understand what I needed to do with my life. Late in her pregnancy, my daughter, Becky, had a fall. Her husband phoned and left a message that she was in the hospital. When I was finally able to call him back, I learned that likely everything would be fine, but I was devastated all the same.

I couldn't go to her because I was scheduled within an inch of my life. I had commitments every day for weeks, and I had never in my life felt so torn in pieces.

Maybe it's a "mother" thing—you hear that the kids are all right, but you won't believe it until you can look them in the eye and see for yourself. Cliff saw how shaken I was as I said to him, "What price are we paying for our success?"

I wanted to go to Becky so much, and I couldn't. Cliff said, "You have to decide what you want to do. If you decide to keep going, I'm behind you. And if you decide to let some of this go, I am with you every step of the way." It was the most stressful moment I'd ever faced, and I did what I knew I had to do.

I started praying immediately. "Lord," I asked, "show me what to do. Make me at peace with my decision." Twenty-four hours later, I knew what I had to do. I realized that I had to go back to the heart and soul of what had become Healthy Exchanges, had to do only what I could do: create recipes, write my books, and keep the newsletter going. I had to let everything else go.

I told myself, if God wants more from me, he'll send help, or he'll show me in some way. Otherwise, my focus was clear: I would concentrate on my family and the creative talent he'd allowed me to share with others.

It was the hardest decision I ever made. Once I made it, it was as if a huge weight was lifted off my heart. The uneasiness was gone. I saw how true it was that stress is a physical thing, and you can actually feel it leave you when you find your true path. I had tried to do so many things, but the energy it had cost me in trying to please people and fulfill promises to everyone had nearly destroyed my life.

I was concerned about the impact my decision would have on others, especially our employees, but I knew I was doing the right thing. As I started to do what I always do—plan and schedule and map out my course of action—I realized it would take about a year to do it all, to get out of or finish up all the commitments I'd already made. We closed the café and did all we could to help people find other jobs, and fortunately their efforts have been successful.

One woman told me she was sorry to be losing her job, but that she'd been wondering how long I could have kept going before I crashed. "It's right," she told me, "right for you and your family." I was touched that she understood, and I appreciated her support, and that of so many others.

In fact, I confess I was surprised by what people said once the news got out. A lot of people told Cliff and me they respected our decision, although they were surprised that such "go-getters" would do it, but they thought it showed more character to step back when things were doing so well.

Their understanding and respect was a real comfort when all kinds of rumors started—that I was dying, that I'd been dropped by my publisher, that I was bankrupt . . . It was disconcerting, to say the least. And closing our business did have some economic implications for our small town. But what got us through those very trying times was knowing we'd made the right decision for us.

It was hard in some ways, putting all the plans we'd made on the shelf. I won't deny there were moments of regret along the way, but when I put them on my mental scale opposite what our decision was giving us as parents, grandparents, and as a couple, we felt more and more sure.

As the weeks and months passed, I came to realize how glad I was that I had stopped on the way up the mountain, before reaching the pinnacle, instead of being on a downward slide. I knew that in ten or fifteen years, life itself would slow me down. I wasn't looking forward to that but, more important, I didn't want my grandkids to ask, "Grandma who?" And when I was old and gray, I didn't want to discover they had no time for me because I'd had no time for them when they were young.

When I first told the kids about my decision, they couldn't have been happier. Becky told me she knew it had been a hard decision for me to make; she'd felt some of the same sorrow when quitting her own business career.

My son James is probably closest to me when it comes to business, since he's such a whiz at marketing and an entrepreneur in his own right, and I think he understood best. He had the most empathy for what the decision would cost me emotionally.

My other son, Tommy, cut to the chase as usual, when he said, "Mom, if you and Cliff are working like dogs to leave the business to us, we'd much rather have your time now than your money later."

I told my family before breaking the news to my employees, and on the day I was ready to make my announcement, the kids were just wonderful. They sent flowers, and the card read, "Congratulations on your decision and enjoy the rest of your life!"

It's been a busy and often chaotic time, but with the downsizing has come an important benefit—much less stress. There are many different ways to measure healthy success, and they aren't all about the bottom line.

Are you stuck in a balancing act that has left you angry,

exhausted, and ready to let your entire china service crash to the floor? I know the feeling all too well! You may think your life is raging out of control, and you don't have a clue what to do about it. Well, here's the good news: By acknowledging that you're aware of the problem, you've already begun to deal with it. Now what's needed is a "Priorities Party"—a chance to sit down with your spouse or kids and talk about what's most important, and what isn't worth it anymore. If you can manage it, set aside time away from home to have this conversation, since trying to cope with a crisis in the middle of Crisis Central might be way too distracting (and you might easily be interrupted, too). This is no time to worry about being objective, either—you're focused on feelings and emotions, your deepest needs as a person, a couple, and a family. Maybe your current financial obligations make second jobs and overtime necessary, but is there a way to scale back without depriving you of what you value most? What would you do if you woke up tomorrow and there was nothing on your "To Do" list? Make a new list called "Wanna Do" instead. After all, if it's what you truly "wanna," then it's vital to find a way.

*Wanna*
*Do List*
*Paint Bench*
*PMP- Classes*
*Painting Class*
*Ceramics*
*Author Conf.*
*Be Slender*
*Be Sexy*
*Dance*

## A Pearl to Polish

*Let your imagination and creativity run wild in coming up with ways to make your "Wanna Do" list real. If you've always dreamed of going back to school but fear you don't have the money or the time, turn it into a family project: research financial aid for returning students, find out more about* distance learning and online classes, figure out how you could adjust your weekly commitments to clear some hours for what's important to you. Instead of accepting what is as what's got to be, imagine your life with those obstacles removed—and see where you'd like to be. It's easier to balance even a busy schedule if the elements in it are those we value most.

# Seeing Yourself As You Are

---

*Most of the important things in the world have been accomplished by people who have kept on trying when there seemed to be no hope at all.*

—DALE CARNEGIE

If I asked you to make a list of the people in your life whose opinions matter to you, where would you begin? Probably with your mother and father, if you're fortunate enough to still have them in your life. Add your spouse or your significant other. Your brothers and sisters, perhaps, or your children. Maybe your boss, and certainly your closest friends.

Think of the people on that list for a moment, and how their opinion of you makes you feel. These people know you in all your many facets, and value you for all the things you are and do. Their good opinion of you has deepened and developed, in most cases, over many years. Their respect and even admiration,

*tough-proof*
*through-*

whether it's for your sensitivity as a parent, your commitment as an employee, or your loyalty as a friend, is based on something real, something meaningful. While I believe your own good opinion of yourself is most important in life, knowing that people we cherish recognize our good qualities surrounds us with a kind of comfort and confidence that sustains us through tough or uncertain times.

I opened a letter recently that got me thinking about this. Marianne's note began, "JoAnna, I feel so worthless when I step on the scale and I've gained a pound. Or even when I've made healthy food choices all week long but I haven't lost an ounce. I have so much weight to lose, and the scale makes me feel like a big, bloated number, not a person. I look in the mirror and I see my weight in big neon-sign numbers, and I'm filled with such disgust. I feel ready to give up on myself and toss that scale in the creek behind my house!"

I know how she feels. I remember how my heart used to just clench when I would climb on the doctor's scale, and they'd have to move those big, heavy weights—200, 250, 300—in order to weigh me. I always hated those sliding scales, having to stand there while the nurse tried to get the scale to balance. And she'd push the little sliding weight up 10 pounds, then 20, 30, 40, 49. . . . It always seemed like such a public humiliation for her to move the next big 50-pound weight into place. My eyes would tear up, and I would find myself wishing I could just sink into the floor and into oblivion.

The scale persuaded me, as it did Marianne, that I was no good. That number, whether it was 150 pounds in my twenties, 225 pounds in my thirties, or 300 pounds in my forties, defined me in a way that made me absolutely miserable. At that moment, the reality that I was a loving daughter, a caring parent, a successful businesswoman, a good friend—none of that mattered. The only opinion I could hear was that of the SCALE—and it told me that I was a big nothing.

*Daughter*

I read a study recently that when you ask a man to describe himself, no matter what his actual measurements and physique, he'll usually smile and say something like, "Well, I've got the same broad shoulders and strong back I had when I played football in high school. I've still got most of my hair, and oh, well, I could stand to lose a few pounds, but my body is pretty good."

That's why I say that positive attitude is more important than any other aspect of living a healthy life. And I don't mean a positive attitude that begins when you reach your goal weight, or one that hinges on hearing your doctor say that your cholesterol count is oh-so-low. A positive attitude about the person in the mirror is maybe the most important tool to getting you where you want to go.

Recently, one of the discussions on my website asked, "What are some of your favorite things about Healthy Exchanges?" I read the responses with interest because I knew each person would have his or her own little victories and moments to cheer, even if they were a long way from reaching their weight-loss and healthy-living goals.

One woman echoed my own experience when she wrote: "I like being able to walk through an airport without being so winded I have to stop to catch my breath every couple of gates. And not having to ask for a seat belt extension is wonderful." Oh, boy, do I remember the humiliation I felt at needing a seat belt extension, and I still recall with pain the number of times I held my hand over the buckle so the flight attendant wouldn't see I needed one. I risked my own life to cover my shame (I'm just grateful I survived without injury), because I couldn't accept that the standard seatbelt wasn't long enough to hold me safely in my seat.

The same woman went on to say how much she liked being able to buy clothes someplace besides out of the large-size catalogs. I always sewed my own clothes, so I didn't suffer through store after store trying to find something in my large size to wear to a family occasion. But so many women have shared with me how hard it was to find self-acceptance when the retail clothing industry refused to make quality clothing in their sizes. (Thank goodness that's less of a problem now. One thing I truly appreciate about QVC is their insistence since Day 1 that designers working for them provide a wide selection of well-made clothing for women up to size 3X. The large sizes are always the first to sell out, so it's clearly good business too!)

But perhaps my favorite line from her note is this: "I like liking myself the way I am today and knowing I can be better tomorrow." YES! For it's only by liking ourselves today that we can work toward our goals of better health. And only by accepting ourselves as we are now can we strive toward a better tomorrow.

Now, I know that it's not easy to admit to liking yourself NOW, when your body is heavier than you'd like it to be. It's much easier to be critical, to be negative and even disgusted by your "extra" flesh. And I'm not saying you have to love and make friends with your poundage, since yes, you are doing all you can to bid it farewell! But you can like who you are as a person without loving absolutely every inch of you. (In fact, you've *got* to, in order to commit to real change!) And loving *who you are* is probably the best first step in learning to love every inch of the healthy body that is your goal!

Most of us have bad memories about seeing ourselves in photographs and discovering just how "fat" we look (or feeling as if we are fat) or how much worse the problem is than we've been willing to believe. But you should know that it's not just overweight people who get depressed about how they look in pictures. Television is a notoriously unflattering medium (they say it puts at least ten pounds on you!), which could explain why the stars of television shows seem to keep getting skinnier and skinner (and scarier and scarier, really!). Those bright lights can make you look older, too—no wonder radio feels less stressful for authors promoting their books!

But seeing yourself as you are isn't just about facing up to how you appear in a store window or a home video. It's more about loving the person inside the flesh, the person of heart and soul who might appear to the world to have a hundred pounds to lose, but who also is intelligent, kind, and dedicated to her career and her family. Accepting yourself, extra pounds and inches and all, is a vital element in developing the kind of positive attitude that delivers long-term results!

I remember reading an article that suggested to people who frequently overate that they sit naked in front of a mirror while dining. (I imagine the advice was geared to single women, as it's tough to imagine propping up a mirror at your kitchen table and gobbling down a sandwich while hoping and praying that your kids or your husband or your mother-in-law didn't show up unannounced!) The idea was that if you could see yourself in the middle of "bad behavior," you'd be so grossed out by your body and your actions that you'd *change*.

The only problem is, disgust and depression aren't really all that motivating, at least not past the first few desperate moments!

And they're not likely to be the ingredients that persuade you to make an enduring lifestyle change. Go on a starvation diet, maybe. Lock yourself in your bathroom and refuse to emerge until you're a size 10, sure. But when you're looking for the kind of encouragement that will sustain you through your struggles to live in a healthier way, demoralizing yourself with such negative images is more likely to backfire. You feel more hopeless than inspired, and you figure that one more cake donut won't make any difference.

The mirror that matters is not the full-length one that hangs on your bedroom wall. It's not the three-way tormentor in the dressing room of your favorite department store. And it's not even the reflection in the eyes of critical friends and relatives.

The mirror that matters most is the one that lets you see inside the skin. It's the magical motivating mirror that tells you that you're not a lost cause, that you're not a hopeless case, that you're not a "loser" in the game of life.

That mirror reflects your true self, the person who has taken on many difficult tasks in life and succeeded in them. That mirror sees what the others can't, that you're a work in progress and not an image frozen in time. If you can learn to accept that vision of yourself, you've got a much better chance to make the physical changes you're working for.

### *A Pearl to Polish*

*What do you like best about the person you see inside your skin? If you were describing yourself to a stranger, and you couldn't use any of the normal physical terms (height, weight, hair color, eye color, etc.), how would you list the qualities and elements that make you distinctively you? Think about a time when you struggled during a conversation with a new acquaintance because you were uncomfortable with your appearance. Now, re-imagine that chat as if the person couldn't see how you looked or how you were dressed. Would you have felt any freer to express your thoughts and feelings? Would the person without sight temporarily see you better without the benefit of his vision? The next time you find yourself in conversation with someone and you're ill at ease because of how you feel about your figure, mentally put a pair of blacked-out sunglasses on the person and keep talking. Soon, you'll be able to do it without the imaginary glasses—and you'll have taken a big step toward seeing yourself as you are.*

# Checking Your Progress
## and Setting Goals

*No dream comes true until you wake up and go to work.*

—ANONYMOUS

*W*hen you make the decision, as I did all those years ago, to change your prayer (and your goal) from simply losing weight (as fast as possible, please!) to recapturing your health and sustaining a healthy lifestyle, it's important to recognize what it means to progress in the direction of your goal. It's too easy to get caught up in what I call "the numbers game"—where what determines your happiness or sorrow, your view of success or failure, happens only on the scale or in your doctor's office. If you see the scale move downward a couple of pounds, joy reigns supreme, but if it stays the same for a week or more, you feel like hiding under the covers! Same thing with the numbers on your blood sugar, your cholesterol, your heart rate monitor. You've been eating healthy for a month or two, or maybe three, and you're expecting a particular result on the test. If the news is all you hoped for, you're delighted, but if you've only accomplished part of your healthy goal, you're ready to quit "because it's not working."

The simple truth is that not all of us progress at the same pace.

Maybe your friend Mary is following the exact same weight-loss plan, and she isn't even exercising as often as you are, but she's lost five more pounds in the past three months. Where's the justice in that?

There just isn't any. I wish I could promise that everyone who dines on Healthy Exchanges recipes and walks for a half hour every day would experience exactly the same success, but I know it's impossible. Every body is different, every person's metabolism operates at a different rate, and each of us is affected by a wide range of factors (age, menstrual cycle for women, medications, genes, past dieting history, and more).

That's why I believe it's important to develop a variety of ways to check your progress, and why it's vital to choose a range of goals that provide motivation and rewards along the way.

What is progress, anyway? Simply put, it means forward movement, but each of us defines that differently. Not all members of a weight-loss support group aspire to fit into a bikini next summer, just as not all people with diabetes aspire to run the Boston Marathon! What makes sense is to establish what represents progress for you—and only you.

I'll never forget when, in the first few months of living a healthier lifestyle, I felt a little thrill while standing at the sink washing out a pair of pantyhose. As I wrung them out and hung them up to dry, I smiled a private little grin that maybe no one but me could truly understand. But I'd just experienced a little victory, a moment of real progress, because when I'd been at my heaviest, a pair of pantyhose never lasted beyond one wearing! Back in 1991, I used to purchase five pair of size-4 extra-large pantyhose every week to wear for work. (At $2.99 a pair, that meant spending $15 a week I would have enjoyed using for something better!) I never knew if my daily pair would even last till quitting time, considering the stress I put on the upper-thigh area.

But long before I reached my goal of losing 130 pounds, I had plenty to celebrate, including the pantyhose victory. I also got to enjoy the Iowa summer months without painful chafing or the private hell of prickly heat, so it really represented three victories in one.

Maybe one of your interim goals (one that has nothing to do with a number on the scale) is something simple, too—carrying your grandchild up the stairs for a diaper change without gasping for breath or fearing you might drop him. Or perhaps it's buttoning the top button on a favorite pair of jeans, or gazing at a photo of yourself without thinking about tearing it to pieces.

What you will find is there are moments in every single day that allow you to mark your progress forward. It's progress when you catch yourself in a negative thought or behavior—and you turn it around to something positive. It's progress when you ask for and get exactly what you want and need in a restaurant at lunch. It's progress when you put down a magazine and lace on your walking shoes because you want to feel the burst of energy that you get from physical activity now. And it's progress when you take the time to plan meals a few days in advance, to organize your pantry for healthy cooking, or to ask a friend what she's serving at a dinner party so you can be sure to have healthy food options, even if it means bringing a dish yourself.

In fact, marking your progress toward better health is one of the most important goals you can set for yourself. It may not seem like it when listed along with bigger dreams, like losing fifty pounds or lowering your blood sugar one hundred points, but learning how to celebrate all the little victories along the way is definitely one of the best tools for actually getting there!

I'm a great believer in setting goals, then doing your best to achieve them, and then setting some new ones. I've used that technique to lose a lot of weight, to grow my business, to cultivate my garden, and to seek balance in my life. I've never felt totally satisfied just resting on my laurels; I like having new horizons to conquer and new dreams just around the bend to pursue. And rather than fixing your gaze and heart on just one faraway goal, I've discovered it's even better to have a plateful of hopes and possibilities to feast on while you "aim for the stars."

Of course, I use that expression carefully, because I also feel it's important to set realistic goals, achievable goals, too. Most of us, at one time or another, have dreamed of looking like movie stars, or winning the lottery, or pitching in the World Series, or raising kids who turn out to be geniuses! But are these obtainable and realistic goals?

In some cases, yes. But perhaps instead of putting all our energies into wishing for such "daydream" goals, it might be worth spending some private time thinking about setting more realistic,

*I need to loose 51,015 LBS.*

"real-world" goals. Losing twenty, fifty, even one hundred pounds, is a realistic goal as long as you don't set an unrealistic time limit. But getting back to the size 7 you wore as a senior in high school—that might not be a realistic goal for you now.

Other realistic goals might include reducing the amount of medication you have to take for high blood pressure, or getting to the point where diet and exercise are sufficient to control your diabetes. A real-world goal might just be dropping one size, from a plus size to a misses' size, so you can shop again in your favorite local boutique. For some of us, a good goal is simply a month, a week, or even a day without feeling powerless in the presence of a plate of cake donuts!

Setting realistic goals means seeing yourself and your life as clearly as possible. Your goals will be different from those of your neighbor, just as your life is different from hers. Don't expect more from yourself than you can realistically give, either. You may feel that nothing less than wearing a size 10 at your daughter's wedding will do. But if God doesn't demand perfection from us, why do we ask it of ourselves? If a wonderful dress in size 12 or 14 makes the mother of the bride look as lovely as her daughter, what difference does the little size tag inside the collar really make?

But don't ask too little of yourself, either. The opposite of chasing perfection is doing little or nothing to improve your life and health, and that's not good enough. So think long and hard about who you are and where you are in your life right now (not ten years ago). Are you basically healthy but need to lose a few pounds? Do you have dangerously high blood pressure in addition to a weight problem? Is your blood sugar controlled by regular injections of insulin or does it frequently skyrocket out of control (especially after a few drinks or an ice cream binge)? Are you comfortably mobile or do you have to use a wheelchair or cane to get around? Do you live in a community where it's safe to walk outside even at night, or are you limited to daylight hours for exercising in the fresh air? Do you even like to walk, or would you rather ride a bike or use a rowing machine? Do you work at home or commute to a distant office? Does caring for your kids make it hard for you to find time to work out before or after a full day at the office?

Before you can begin to set realistic goals, you need to be honest with yourself about what limitations or challenges your lifestyle imposes on you. Can you work to change some of those limitations? Certainly, especially over time, but aiming right away for a goal that requires a major shift in your daily life might be setting yourself up for failure. An example of that might be deciding to join a gym near your home, without accepting the reality that your long commute means leaving the house at 7 A.M. and returning close to 9 P.M. each day. A more realistic fitness goal might be signing up for a lunchtime exercise class near your office instead.

Figuring out where you are is the first step on the road to getting where you want to go. You're starting at Point A, and you want to arrive at Point B, but you've got a number of possible routes to consider. You aren't going to cover the entire distance in a day or even a week, so dividing the "mileage" into manageable segments is also part of planning for a safe, fun, and successful journey. And just as you would pack the car with snacks and distractions to help pass the time, so too should you include those items in your "pretrip" planning!

The same is true when it comes to setting healthy lifestyle goals. Since extra poundage can cause all kinds of health concerns, the opposite is also true: losing excess weight, or even a portion of it, can provide immediate health benefits. But since the experts and professionals suggest that a slow, steady weight loss is best for your body over time, you want to think reasonably about what your goal should be.

First, you decide that the goal is to lose twenty-five pounds. Let's assess the goal: Is it too much or too little for your height and body type? After visiting with a doctor, meeting with a registered dietitian, or reviewing a reputable weight chart that takes into consideration age, sex, build, and activity level, you determine that it's an appropriate goal.

Now, the professional dieter I used to be would have checked out the latest diet fad—probably a liquid or pill or unproven supplement—and decided that if it could "melt" the weight off in a month or six weeks, it was perfect for my needs. But I'm not looking to race along the weight-loss Interstate at twenty miles over the speed limit anymore. I know the odds for safety aren't in my favor, and I also know that I'd likely be doomed to travel down that same road again. So I recommend setting a different goal this time, just like the tortoise who ultimately beat the hare—"slow but steady wins the race"—and planning to follow a sensible eating plan that is likely to take off that twenty-five pounds in about a year at the rate of about a half pound per week. Since we all know that some weeks you may not lose anything, and other weeks a pound may happily "fall off," this plan offers a reasonable hope of meeting that goal in that time.

How can you help yourself meet that long-term goal? By

choosing a food plan you can stick with, one that doesn't ask you to deprive yourself in the short term or over time. By making time for exercise that will burn additional calories. By working to establish healthy habits and positive behaviors that will sustain you through the tough times and for the rest of your life.

Breaking a goal into smaller segments is always a good idea, because it gives you more opportunities for celebration. A recent e-mail shared Jenny's ongoing weight-loss journey in this way: "I'm enjoying reaching all kinds of goals, and rewarding myself with new fitness videos, great padded walking socks, and pretty ponytail holders for my daily walks," she wrote. "Each five pounds, of course, but also the round numbers on the scale. Because I started at 227, I rewarded myself for reaching 5 pounds off (222), reaching 220, reaching 10 pounds off (217), reaching 215, and so on. Now I'm at 192, and celebrating 35 pounds down, but also looking forward to going below 190. All these interim goals give me a boost toward the next, and when the scale is a little sluggish, I just focus on how good I feel about how far I've come!"

Jenny noted some other goals that meant as much to her as the downward movement of the scale. "I'm running again, not a whole mile yet, but for longer chunks of distance each time I head out. And yesterday I did a step aerobics workout and for the first time I used two risers to lift the step up. It was harder, but I was still able to do the whole tape. I remember when I struggled to finish the workout without any risers at all!"

But what really made me smile was her final comment, because it hit home for me, too. She wrote, "It's a good thing I live alone, JoAnna, because I am always looking in the mirror and smiling at myself. I can see the changes in my face and in my body, and I love how I look. I've still got lots to lose, but all the positive reinforcement I get from checking myself out is keeping me motivated!"

Whatever your goals are, and no matter how small they might seem, write them down and work in small and bigger ways toward reaching them. You might be the only person who cares that your arms have grown stronger from lifting weights and so you can now French-braid your hair without taking breaks to rest. You may be the only person who notices that your clavicle bones are visible when you wear a V-neck sweater. Whether it's walking a mile two minutes faster this month than last month, or fitting into a dress you wore on your honeymoon, it's a worthwhile goal—worth noting and worth celebrating. In my book *Make a Joyful Table,* I wrote that we need to celebrate more as we grow older and life is infinitely more precious. Don't wait for the big victories to strike up the band—acknowledge yourself today!

### A Pearl to Polish

*A wise person once said, "Begin where you are. But don't stay where you are." Begin by believing that you can accomplish what you wish to do. Begin each day by reminding yourself what is truly important to you, and then start moving in that direction.*

# The Perfect Day

*If you wait for the perfect moment when all is safe and assured, it may never arrive. Mountains will not be climbed, races won, or lasting happiness achieved.*

—MAURICE CHEVALIER

If every day were perfect, it would be perfectly wonderful, wouldn't it? But needless to say, that's not how life really is. Sometimes we wake up in the morning with our entire day planned, only to have everything go awry before we even get to the breakfast table. But we can daydream about what a perfect day would be like, can't we?

Let me tell you about My Perfect Day:

- I wake up at 5 A.M. because *I want to,* not because I have to.
- The day promises to be 72 degrees and sunny, with a southerly breeze and not a rain cloud in sight.

- I walk two miles without any interruptions from barking dogs, low-flying birds, or passing cars and trucks.
- We didn't run out of skim milk the night before, so I can enjoy a cold glass with my breakfast.
- I have time to do a load of laundry and tidy up the house before I start work.
- The morning paper arrives early, so I have time to read more than Ann Landers.
- I am at my desk by 7 A.M., and by some miracle (elves in the night?) it is not its normal cluttered mess.
- I write at my computer for at least two hours, uninterrupted, and I get more words spelled right than wrong.
- I do a couple of radio interviews by phone so that I can share my "common folk" healthy recipes and common-sense approach to healthy living with others.
- I create and test a couple of new recipes, and they turn out right the very first time.
- I manage to answer all my pending correspondence: letters, e-mails, and faxes.
- My grandkids come to visit and I get tons of hugs and kisses from them, but they leave before any diapers need to be changed!
- I tend to my gardens for at least an hour, digging and weeding and watering to my heart's content.
- Not a single cross word is spoken between Cliff and me as the day unfolds.
- Each of my three children calls me sometime during the day just to say hi.

- I stop work by 6:30 P.M., ride my bike for at least two miles to unwind, prepare supper using more test recipes, do some pleasure reading, watch a little TV with Cliff, and call it a night by 10 P.M., so I can dream visions of another perfect day.

How many of my days are even close to being this perfect? *Not very many!* But here's some food for thought on the subject: The greatest baseball players of all are thrilled with a batting average of .300, which means that for every three times they come to bat, they only get a hit once. So I guess if I can have at least four to six of the items on my Perfect Day list on any given day, then I'll remain reasonably content. And those few glorious days when everything falls into place—I'll just consider them as special blessings from God, and not expect every single day to be perfect.

What's the object of all this, you may wonder? Well, if you don't know what you want out of your life, how can you know if you are getting it? If you've never given any substantial thought to what makes a Perfect Day from your point of view, how can you include as much perfection as possible in your very best days?

So—why not take a few minutes now and jot down your idea of a Perfect Day? Be sure to ask yourself what makes you happiest in all areas of your life, from your home and family to your job and leisure-time activities. Don't use this exercise as an excuse to list only what you think you should include; instead, live "dangerously" and list only what is truly pleasing for you. What do I mean by that? Well, if you're not especially happy in your job, then your Perfect Day is probably a day off, but perhaps there is a message in that that could direct you toward a search for a new, more fulfilling kind of work at some near or distant time. If your Perfect Day includes spending time with children but you're single at the moment, you could envision a time when you're married with kids of your own, but you could also create an "in-the-meantime" way to volunteer on a pediatric ward or pick up some extra cash baby-sitting.

Don't think too hard or long about this, or you'll tend to censor yourself, including what you think you should instead of what you dream about. Okay, now that you've got your list in front of you, how are you doing? Batting .300 or better most of the time? Then I hope you are offering prayers of thanks that your life is so close to being exactly what you want it to be.

Some things, of course, are out of our control, like the weather, so if you relish tropical breezes and you live in frequently drizzly Seattle, then you may only get your Perfect Day weather on vacation in Hawaii. (Of course, you could dream a Perfect Day vision that sets as one of your "someday" goals a retirement home in a warm climate. . . .) But we can take charge of many of our own circumstances, some as small as remembering to purchase a new container of milk when it gets down to halfway empty, or by not overextending ourselves by committing to more than we have time to do and do well.

Even though the letter *P* is the last letter in the word *HELP,* I consider it the most important. (Doesn't the Bible tell us, the last shall be first?) That *P* is for Positive Attitude, and I believe that everything else good that we do for ourselves and others comes from the power it provides. Part of Positive Attitude is learning to rejoice in the simple pleasures of life, even tiny things like the song of a bird while I'm riding along a country road or the warmth in my daughter's voice when Becky calls to tell me my grandchild's latest accomplishment!

Since I made my own Perfect Day list, I've come to appreciate how fortunate I really am. I get to do what I love best, I get to share it with others, I'm blessed with a wonderful family and a terrific partner in life and work . . . You know, I might just be rising to the top of the Major League of Life, I've got so many things to be thankful for! Some weeks, I've realized, I'm batting .400, even .500, and those good times help me through the tougher ones.

Keep your Perfect Day list next to your bed or in your desk drawer. Update it and revise it from time to time, but keep it in mind. If you're not batting at least .300 now, try to figure out where you can "improve your average" and start enjoying your daily life to the fullest! You'll be glad you did.

### *A Pearl to Polish*

*Your ideas about "perfection" are likely to change from year to year. Recognize that what looks perfect in your mind's eye may turn out to be much less than ideal if and when it is ever achieved. So—rethink it! The sooner we accept that none of us is perfect, the easier it is to move from harsh self-criticism to positive attitude and self-love. Here's an idea: Think of someone in your life whose imperfections get on your nerves, and focus instead on what is best in that person. Once you train yourself to find the good in what you tend to see as bad in someone else, you'll see how much easier it gets to take pleasure and satisfaction in your own little victories.*

# Managing Motivation

---

*The Constitution only gives people the right to pursue happiness. You have to catch it yourself.*

—BENJAMIN FRANKLIN

Whenever I have a speaking engagement, I schedule a question-and-answer session as part of the event. I can almost guarantee that every single time, someone is bound to ask me, "Yes, but how do you stay motivated?" (I wish I had a quarter for each one—I'd have an overflowing piggy bank!)

Even though I've heard this question a zillion times now, I know that it's as immediate a concern to the woman in front of me as it has been to thousands of others over the past decade. *Motivation* is the word we all use when we're looking for staying power, something we hope will keep us moving in the right direction, some magic trick to make the hard times easy and the effort less of a challenge. When we're motivated, we know what to do and we do it, without a struggle. And when we lose our motivation, we lose more than our way—we accept failure, and we slide back to a place of unhappiness and unhealthiness.

What is this thing called motivation, and why is it often so short-lived and unreliable? Is there some kind of psychological trick we can pull out of a hat when our determination wavers and our commitment weakens? Is the notion of motivation a dangerous one, since it implies something you have when you succeed and something don't have when you fail?

There's no easy answer to any of these questions, just a myriad of life experience and hard-earned understanding of how our hearts and minds work. Even though I've managed to lose 130 pounds and keep it off for nearly a decade now, I'm no miracle worker—and I'm not Saint JoAnna either. I'm just a middle-aged working wife, mother, and grandmother who figured out a few answers that helped me lighten up. Now I look forward to waking up each morning so I can *do it all over again!*

But while I don't have any magic tricks up my sleeve, I'm happy to share what I've discovered about getting and staying motivated on my own journey toward healthy living and self-acceptance. Some of what worked for me may strike a chord for you, or it may at least get you thinking about what might help you create and reach for your own goals. There's no one solution to this eternal question, but fortunately there are many possibilities that could be the answer you're looking for!

When we're young and struggling with a weight problem, motivation may be a simple matter—you want to fit into a particular pair of jeans, or you've got a dance coming up and your heart is set on something strapless and short. As you get older, a better appearance continues to be a goal, but you've also learned a few things about how your habits may impact your health, especially over the long term. Maybe your father discovers a heart problem or your mother is diagnosed as a diabetic; perhaps a close friend begins taking medication to reduce cholesterol or lower blood pressure. Suddenly, you're not just worried about how you look but also about how you feel—and how you're going to feel for the rest of your life.

The word *motivation,* by the way, has a Latin root that means "to move," and so far we've discovered that you can be *moved* by a desire to look better and by the fear that your health is endangered. These concerns encourage you to move from where you are to where you want to be. You're motivated—but will the spirit that moves you in the direction of better health stay strong and unyielding when something else "moves" you—say, the desire to party with friends and gobble down fast food and a few beers, or the fear of not fitting in because you've chosen not to drink or smoke?

It took me until I was in my forties to find my true motivation. It took a time of real personal crisis for me to recognize that what I'd found was a whole new way of thinking. The date was January 4, 1991, at 9:05 A.M., when I changed my goal from simply losing weight to recapturing my health. My children were away defending our nation, and I was faced with a bigger concern than the size of my hips or my appetite. Would they survive? Would I become a burden to them because of the physical problems I faced by being so dangerously overweight? I found what had been missing up to that point: motivation to change. When I decided to start living a HELP lifestyle (though I hadn't named it yet), I realized I was no longer willing to keep doing the crazy things to my spirit and body that I'd somehow forced myself to endure for the length of my latest DIET. I started treating myself with a kind of dignity and respect, recognizing that I was a person of value no matter what size my waist was. Instead of being motivated by feelings of disgust or self-loathing, I took a positive attitude—and found the strength to do what I needed to take care of myself. Positive thinking became a part of my everyday life, and the little acts of kindness I did for myself started to reap huge harvests!

How could something as vague as "kindness" make all the difference, especially to a woman who weighed more than three hundred pounds? It's something you'll have to take on faith until you try it for yourself. But think for a moment how it feels to look in the mirror and hate what you see in there. Think how it feels to struggle to zip up a pair of size-28 pants that you know are too tight, although you can't bring yourself to shop for bigger ones. Think how it feels to make a hearty casserole for your family, then nibble melba toast and cottage cheese for your own dinner. Think how it feels to have to move the seat in the car so far back you can barely reach the gas pedal just so you can buckle your seatbelt. Think how it feels never to eat dessert in front of anyone. Think how it feels to have to have your wedding ring cut off because your fingers become too swollen for you to wear it. Any or all of these "for instances" are part of the daily existence of many overweight people, and it's easy to understand how each one isolates and embitters the person who experiences it. And treating yourself with kindness is definitely not the first thing that comes to mind. Self-criticism is much more likely; self-loathing is much more common. Neither of these, of course, is apt to help you make changes for the better.

But kindness—kindness is more powerful than you know. Kindness begins with acceptance of *what is.* Kindness means focusing on what you like about yourself in the mirror—shiny hair, beautiful complexion, pretty eyes. Kindness could mean picking up a button extension in the sewing store so you can fasten your slacks more easily, or easing the waistband with an insert of elastic. Kindness to yourself is committing to making a tasty low-fat casserole for dinner that you can enjoy with your family. Kindness is choosing to view the world like the fictional character of Pollyanna, who used to play the Glad Game, finding something in every situation to be glad about. (I confess it, my family used to call me Joeyanna, so this notion is close to my heart!)

I realized on that cold January day that each dawn is a new treasure, a gift of twenty-four hours to live life to the fullest and the healthiest we possibly can. And I discovered, quite to my amazement, that when you are filled with positive attitude, eating cake donuts and lying around like a couch potato soon lose their appeal.

Even from the very beginning, I thought about motivation, and about ways to keep myself moving in the right direction. I decided to reward myself for **little deeds** and they soon grew into **large feats.** I applauded myself for every small positive change I made in my life, not just with encouraging comments, but with actual reminders of what I had done. These rewards weren't just tied to the numbers on the scale, either, but also to the positive actions I was taking in my life, from making time to exercise to substituting other activities for unconscious snacking to stopping myself in mid-thought or comment when negative words reared their ugly heads!

Once I became my own best friend, I saw firsthand how my

positive attitude was changing my life in every possible way. Cutting remarks or jokes from others about my weight no longer triggered a desire to retaliate with a burst of "I'll show them" even-more-out-of-control eating. I knew I was doing the best I could . . . *the best I could,* even if others couldn't see it yet.

Yet even after all these years I haven't forgotten how hurt I felt when a co-worker penetrated my "shield" of positive attitude. On my last day of work as a commercial insurance underwriter (before I left to devote my energies full-time to Healthy Exchanges), this "friend" sat down at my desk, looked me in the eye, and with a smirk on her face asked, "But JoAnna, what are you going to do *when* you gain all your weight back?" It was hard not to succumb to a mountain of self-doubt in that moment, but only my daily reinforcement of positive attitude got me through that moment (and some other tough ones over the years). I know now with a confidence I didn't have back then that my hard work and healthy habits will help keep me from having to answer that "loaded" question. Fueled by positive thoughts, I'm stronger than those who would seek to discourage me. That's the first of my secrets I want to share with you!

I even found a way to apply positive attitude to exercise by turning what could have become a daily chore into a fun game with me as the guaranteed winner. Each year, I walk from DeWitt, Iowa, to New York City. Each year, I ride my bike from DeWitt all the way to Los Angeles, California. Every day, even if I walk only a mile or pedal just two or three, I mark off the distance on a map and know that I am moving toward a goal. (Motivation = moving, remember!) When I've traveled enough miles to stand on the Brooklyn Bridge or ride along Rodeo Drive, I reward myself with a nonfood treat that celebrates my accomplishment. Cake donuts aren't good enough anymore to reward me for what I've done! Instead, I choose something that has a special meaning only to me. I've selected plants for my garden, pretty costume jewelry to lend a little sparkle to my jackets, wall plaques with sayings that give me a little positive boost when I glance up at them. Nothing is very expensive, but I don't shop at the dime store either. I want my "trophies" to last, so that every time I look at them, I can remember the occasion that allowed me to earn that reward.

One woman I know chose a silver ankle bracelet for her exercise accomplishment. "As I walk fast around the neighborhood, it slithers just a little up and down my leg," she told me. "I feel just a little sexy wearing it, and I like knowing it's my gift to myself for reaching the first twenty-five pounds of my weight-loss goal!"

I also hold a yearly Reward Ceremony Day, and I'm the only invited recipient at the annual celebration. I've chosen to celebrate the anniversary of when I decided to live healthy instead of dieting. I call it my "Healthy Living Anniversary." So every January 4, I weigh myself, and as long as I weigh the same or less than the year before, and as long as I'm living in a healthy way, I reward myself with an attractive ring. Now that I'm no longer obsessed with dieting, I've been able to reward myself every year since that fateful day in 1991. In my old yo-yo dieting days, I would have been lucky if I'd maintained my weight loss for a month, let alone all these years! Besides my wedding ring, I now wear all my "reward" rings on the fingers of both hands. Every time I need a quick fix of positive motivation, all I have to do is glance down at my hands, admire those rings, and say to myself, "Good job, JoAnna!" (Cliff jokes that I'll have to start wearing more than one ring per finger pretty soon, or else grow another pair of hands.) Now that my fingers are filled, and each ring is too important to me to take off, I've changed my reward to paintings for my wall. But I know one thing for sure, that I'll continue to celebrate my "Healthy Living Anniversary" date and reward myself for the rest of my life.

That's another of my secrets for staying motivated, for continuing to *move* in the right direction. But motivation is very personal, and you will have to discover what sparks your spirit and moves you to keep going where you want to be. One of my readers promised herself a "glamour" photo session when she got down to her goal weight and firmed up her body through her exercise classes. Another wanted to run a local 10-kilometer race in under an hour. Still another wanted to have a second child but felt that she was more likely to have a healthy pregnancy if she lost some weight and got her high blood pressure under control first.

All these goals are wonderful, and they can have an amazing power to motivate you. But what happens when you reach your goals? What becomes of your motivation then? Most of us have managed to lose weight throughout our dieting lives, but keeping it off was the test we couldn't seem to pass. That's one of the reasons I believe in having more than one goal to sustain motivation, so that celebrating your success doesn't work against you instead of for you. I think that's one reason my anniversary works for me—because the goal is lifelong, and focuses on getting somewhere *and* staying there.

Sometimes what works is a list of goals you add to each year, or each time you reach one and get to cross it off. Maybe a goal for the coming year is learning something new—the tango, how to drive a stick shift, how to use a new computer program. Not all your goals have to be weight- or exercise-related; healthy living celebrates the mind as much as it does the body. The secret seems to be in the notion of motion—keep moving forward, keep learning and growing and changing. It's another way of thinking positively—finding ways to add to the wonderful person you are.

If you're struggling to find what moves you, if motivation seems elusive right now, don't focus on the big picture for the moment. Start with the coming week. Take a few minutes each day and pat yourself on the back for anything positive you do. Keep a little notebook where you list each of these little victories, and don't deny yourself a celebratory moment because the item seems too insignificant to record. If you make time in a busy day to go on a short walk at lunchtime, **write it down**. If twice this week (instead of not at all) you prepare a complete meal using all healthy recipes, **write it down**. If you handle a stressful situation without resorting to old habits or reaching for unhealthy comfort foods to "make it all better," **write it down.** At the end of the week, take a few minutes to read everything you've written, and if you're like most of us, I bet you'll be surprised at *all the things you do right!*

Every day is a new opportunity to do what makes you feel good. Every day provides another chance to reinforce the healthy habits you've decided are important to you. Just keep doing the best you can. . . . *the best you can,* even if you're the only one who notices. Before you know it, everyone will notice the changes in you. Then they'll start asking you, "Yes, but how do you stay motivated?" Smile, and share your secrets, beginning with kindness and encouragement. There's never too much positive attitude in the world, don't you agree?

## *A Pearl to Polish*

*Journalist Susan L. Taylor, whose vision shaped* Essence *magazine, wrote, "Seeds of faith are always within us; sometimes it takes a crisis to nourish and encourage their growth." Each time you struggle to sustain the changes you've made in yourself, each time you consider the possibility of returning to old, self-destructive behaviors and you find the courage to stick to your new path, you are expressing your faith in yourself and in the journey you've chosen.*

# Chill Out!

———

*Finish each day and be done with it. You have done what you could. Some blunders and absurdities no doubt crept in; forget them as soon as you can. Tomorrow is a new day; begin it well and serenely and with too high a spirit to be cumbered with your old nonsense.*

—RALPH WALDO EMERSON

*S*tress can do a lot more than cause worry wrinkles around your eyes. It can be a contributing factor to heart problems; it can cause blood sugar levels to reach sky-high; and for many of us, it's a major trigger for overeating and weight gain.

If you are constantly under pressure, coping with anxiety, dealing with people or things that upset you, your body knows it. And when things get out of control, the results can be a dozen different health concerns.

Did you know that stress can cause poor judgment and rash reactions to problems that arise? (Imagine being super stressed-out

*[handwritten margin notes: MY Stress-causes; Upset Stomach; Insomnia; Fatigue; Headach]*

and having to cope with a reckless driver coming way too close to your car!)

Did you know that stress can cause an inability to concentrate, chronic irritability, stomach cramps, diarrhea, insomnia, elevated blood pressure, backaches—shall I stop there? (Just typing that list was stressful enough!)

Did you know that stress is linked to excessive smoking, to alcohol abuse, and to overeating? (I bet you did.)

Now, did you notice that the problems stress causes are both physical and emotional? Stress can play a powerful role in all kinds of physical and psychological maladies, and the long-term effects of coping (or not coping) with the stress in your life can be terrible.

Here's the thing about stress: You have a lot more control than you may know over how much stress you allow in your life, and how you react to the stress you're faced with every day. Everyone seems to agree that life in the twenty-first century is more hectic than in the past. Sure, we've got millions of time-saving appliances and computerized this-and-thats, but the problem is something the techies call "multi-tasking." What that means is we're trying to cram more activities into the day than we have time for, all in the name of being efficient. (Why, of course, you can answer your e-mail while talking on the phone to your mother and gobbling down a lukewarm microwaved entree!)

The question is, what price are we paying for all that efficiency and accomplishment? Are we destroying our bodies and driving our minds to the edge in the name of getting "things" done? Maybe it's time, as they used to say, to CHILL OUT!

When the daily demands of life overwhelm you and you're feeling exhausted, angry, and just this side of crazy, the last thing you want to do is add to the burden you're shouldering by overeating, or by taking it out on those around you. Instead, why not reach for one of the following commonsense suggestions. They've helped me cope with stressed-out times, and perhaps they will help you and the people about whom you care most.

- **Identify the source of your stress.** Is it a person who turns your entire office into a toxic environment? Is it a friend who's going through her own problems but lately has been pawning them off on you? Is it a spouse who's not doing his or her part to keep the family running smoothly? Is it a child who turns every breakfast into a battleground over everything from food to friends to fashion? Once you've identified the source, try to find positive, practical ways of changing the situation. It may be painful to confront the problem head-on, but the alternative is sacrificing your own physical and mental health.

- **When you have scheduled appointments—dentist, hairdresser, your child's teacher—leave enough time to get ready and to get there.** I wonder if anyone's done a study of how many traffic accidents are caused by stressed-out drivers who are late for an appointment, and whose common sense goes out the window when all they can hear is the clock ticking! So make it easier on yourself—allow extra time for unexpected heavy traffic. (One woman I spoke with actually "tricks" herself by subtracting fifteen minutes from the actual time of the appointment when she writes it in her calendar. She heads for a 3 P.M. doctor's appointment "believing" that it's at 2:45, so she can breathe easier—and leave the office a few minutes earlier, too). If you're dealing with a spouse or child who is frequently late, try this little "trick" on them. "Dinner's at 6:15," you remind your husband, knowing that you're expecting to serve at 6:30. While this technique won't teach them to be on time (and you may feel that the struggle isn't worth it), it will help get them there when you want them to be, and keep your own temper from reaching the boiling point!

- **Count to ten or, better yet, take a short walk before reacting to a stressful situation.** It's almost always best to delay your response until you can calmly review all the facts and make a clearheaded decision. Acting impulsively is risky, and it often encourages you to say things in anger you'd rather not have said, just making things worse. By taking a few extra minutes, by catching your breath and considering your options, you remove some of the situation's "heat" and reduce the physical and emotional anguish on your body.

- **Learn to compromise.** Give in occasionally. Does the family room always need to be spotless? Why not let someone who's signaling frantically enter the traffic lane in front of you for once? How about letting your "significant other" have the last word sometimes? Compromise doesn't mean being a doormat or a slouch. Instead, it suggests that not every issue deserves a full-fledged battle, that not every occasion requires you to be the first, the best, the winner. It's also about sharing control, even surrendering it some of the time. Maybe you *are* a better driver than your spouse, but sometimes it's okay just to sit back and enjoy the view. And yes, you could have organized the bake sale more efficiently than the committee who did, but think of how much less time you'd have had to spend with your kids last weekend, and besides, it's enough that you contributed a Triple Layer Party Pie!

- **Do little things that make a big difference.** In many homes, stress levels rise whenever someone can't find the car keys or the house keys or stamps for an overdue bill to be mailed. Why not designate a special place where these items can "live" and never go astray again—a handy homemade key rack, a sturdy bowl on a hall table, a drawer in your sewing table to hold all your stationery supplies? If the main stress producer in your house is always running out of "necessaries" or forgetting to refill the gas tank, make a rule that as soon as the orange juice carton is half empty, OJ goes on the shopping list, and as soon as the gas tank shows a quarter tank, it gets filled by the next person to drive the car.

- **Pay attention to what you put in your mouth.** Prepare for stressful times by having healthy snacks ready and waiting—low-fat granola bars, small bags of Wow! potato chips, pop-top cans of fruit, or whatever works for you. The worst thing you can do when you're exhausted is fill yourself with unhealthy foods that deliver empty calories and none of the healthful energy you really need to cope. By always stocking your fridge and cupboard with the foods you need for a nourishing menu, you'll lower your stress level every time you enter the kitchen. Besides, if your goal is losing weight and keeping it off, eating junk will only produce greater stress!

- **Stop procrastinating.** If you know you have to do something that you've been putting off, do it today, or make a very specific plan to do it as soon as possible. You'll feel so relieved that it's done, your stress level will shoot way down, and you won't have to wake up every day with the black cloud of an approaching deadline hanging over your head. If you need encouragement to get to it, figure out an appropriate (and not unhealthy) "bribe"—a hot bath before bedtime, or a new paperback mystery to read when the "assignment" is completed.

- **Give your spouse, your kids, your grandkids, and anyone else who is important to you impromptu hugs and kisses.** Don't wait for a special occasion to express affection for the people you love, and don't be a miser with it, either! Your loving touch is as good for you as it is for the lucky recipient. I've even read that the body produces endorphins—feel-good chemicals—at such times, driving the stress level way, way down. If you don't have anyone nearby to hug, cuddle your cat, and if you don't have a live creature to lavish affection on, I've been told that you're never old to hug a teddy bear!

- **Last, but certainly not least, realize that some things are just not under your control.** (Oh, did you think that you were in charge of the world and everything in it?) That old Serenity Prayer reminds us to change the things we can, but also to recognize that some things are beyond our control. Wisdom, and yes, a lot less stress, comes in recognizing the difference and making our peace with it. Take charge where you can, make changes if you're able, but learn to let go of anything you can't influence or shape to your satisfaction. People are amazingly hard to change. You and your father-in-law will never agree on tax reform? Then make a vow not to engage in exhausting, angry discussions on the topic. Just smile and say, "Oh well, let's agree to disagree on that one." You used to love arranging flowers for the church on Sunday mornings, but you're tired of the arguments between the others on the committee? Maybe it's time to resign and put your positive energy to use in some other way—the choir? teaching Sunday school? or just spending more time with your own family before services begin? What feels like surrender isn't. You're making a choice for your health and your sanity, and it's a victory instead.

### *A Pearl to Polish*

*Stress is most often the result of a conflict—between how we see the world and how we wish it would be. But the mental and physical anguish that accompanies stress doesn't help us change the world for the better. Instead, it makes us less able to cope with what is. Just for today, consider just one thing that raises your blood pressure and makes your stomach churn. Accept that it exists, and figure out a way around this obstacle that makes you come out a healthy winner!*

# Listening to and
# Learning from Others

*I am always ready to learn although I do not always like being taught.*

—WINSTON CHURCHILL

$\mathcal{D}$o you sometimes feel that you are the only person who has to pass up tempting sweets, or make time for exercise when everyone else is relaxing in front of the TV, nibbling away on crunchy goodies?

Do you change your plans because you're worried how you'll handle every special occasion, every holiday party, or every family gathering that involves food?

Do you allow your frustration and isolation to build up until you want to shout to the heavens, "Why me?"

Even if it feels that way, you're not alone.

In fact, you've got a lot of company just about everywhere. You may think you're the only one who has to choose carefully from among the buffet dishes, but if you turn your attention away from yourself for a moment, you may notice that your cousin Harry (a recently diagnosed diabetic) is gazing longingly at the banana cream pie, or that your new neighbor from down the street is drinking club soda instead of alcohol at the block party. If you are willing to delve a bit deeper, you might learn that your PTA committee chairwoman has been warned by her doctor to make a lot of lifestyle changes or face being put on blood pressure medication for the rest of her life. You might even discover that the principal's wife, whom you've always envied for her beautiful appearance, is quietly battling breast cancer and hiding her hair under a scarf until it grows back.

It's very common, especially when you're focusing your attention on recapturing your own health, to turn so completely inward that you lose perspective. All you can think about is how a situation affects you, whether it's figuring out what to eat at a dinner party or squeezing in a half-hour walk when you're traveling with your kids. It's fine to carve out time for yourself—in fact, it's a necessity—but when you begin to grow impatient because of the effort required to live consciously and make healthy choices, you may develop a case of "Why me?" You may find yourself asking, "Why do I have to eat grilled fish when everyone else is having fried chicken? Why am I alone on New Year's Eve when the rest of the world is paired up and having fun? Why? Why ? Why? Why? Why?"

Does that sound like anyone you know? It's the kind of attitude that some people develop when they grow tired of "being good," fed up with "behaving themselves," or annoyed with the speed at which they're losing weight or regaining their health.

But it's a self-defeating attitude that has real consequences, because you may convince yourself that it's not fair, that you deserve a break from your diet, that exercise isn't all it's cracked up to be. Before you know it, you're back in the rut of bad habits that made you want and need to change in the first place!

One of the ways you can stay grounded in the real world is by listening to and learning from others in the same boat. That requires a conscious effort to tune in to what other people are experiencing, to consider what they're feeling, and to offer ideas and options to help keep them on track. The payoff comes in two ways: first, you know that you're not the only one struggling, moaning, or feeling frustrated; and second, you're in a position to boost their spirits, and by doing so, give your own a shot in the arm!

Every time I go out on a book tour or get a chance to meet my readers when I'm judging at the Iowa State Fair or speaking at a convention, I notice that while people are waiting to visit with me, they start sharing with each other, and the very first tentacles of friendship begin stretching out between them. They may have come to listen and learn from me, but they're getting more than they bargained for. Each person engaged in the journey to better health is a resource, and his or her experiences have value for others who meet them. Dr. George Sheehan, the running doctor who wrote so many inspiring columns that had more to do with living well than running faster, once said, "Each of us is an experiment of one." I think he meant that we may learn from ourselves what the experts in the field have not yet encountered in their research. Instead of keeping what we learn to ourselves, it makes sense to share our knowledge, our inspirations, and our hopes with others walking the same path.

If you've chosen to attend a support group for weight loss or diabetes management, then you've got a built-in community already. If you're working on cardiac rehab at a gym or working out with friends, you can start there to listen and learn—and when you're ready, to share.

But what if you're homebound because of illness, or you're taking care of young children and find it hard to get out of the house? What if the only free time you can find is after midnight, when everyone has gone to sleep and it's just you and the computer? Well, welcome to the New World, Ms. and Mr. Columbus, because your colleagues and comrades are just a "click" away!

When we began the Healthy Exchanges website (healthyexchanges.com), I thought it would be a good way to share my story, promote and sell my cookbooks, and perhaps make it easier to reach readers when Cliff and I were on the road. What I didn't understand at the time was how powerful this site and others like it could become in just a few short months. Because, in addition to those other goals, we've made it possible for people to listen to and learn from each other through message boards and even nightly chats. Some who've met on the boards have gone on to build e-mail friendships; a few, who discovered they were nearly neighbors, have even arranged to meet face-to-face!

I've always tried to listen to and learn from my readers. From the very start, I wanted them to know that we were all in this together. They're the reason I created the many reader feedback sections in my newsletters. The same has been true for the website. Occasionally I like to peek in and read the posts, to find out how people feel about the recipes I've created and how they've incorporated my suggestions into a healthy lifestyle.

But I've also been very moved by how generous people are when it comes to helping each other. Those who are following a weight-loss program but perhaps not attending regular meetings have a chance to experience truly welcoming group support. Those who are struggling with the decision to begin again receive encouragement from people they barely know but whose words can be surprisingly powerful. As the months have passed, I've been touched by all kinds of stories—deeply satisfying tales of weight lost and health regained, painful reports of unkind remarks that the writer felt free to share only with her online buddies, intimate confessions of coping with the loss of a spouse or the challenges of a disability without finding solace in binge eating or other destructive behavior.

With the permission of the writers, I am able to share two posts that caught my eye as I was working on this book. I was deeply touched by what each correspondent wrote in response to the needs of the others visiting the website.

The first came during the holiday season from Carolyn of Texas, who responded with sensitivity when she felt that some of her online friends were "sad and feeling blue and alone at this time." She wrote,

Here is my wish for you:

Your presence is a present to the world. You're unique and one of a kind. Your life can be what you want it to be. Take the days just one at a time.

Count your blessings, not your troubles. You'll make it through whatever comes along. Within you are so many answers. Understand, have courage, be strong.

Don't put limits on yourself. So many dreams are waiting to
be realized. Decisions are too important to leave to
chance. Reach for your peak, your goal, your prize.

Nothing wastes more energy than worrying. The longer one
carries a problem, the heavier it gets. Don't take things
too seriously. Live a life of serenity, not a life of regrets.

Remember that a little love goes a long way. Remember
that a lot . . . goes forever. Remember that friendship
is a wise investment. Life's treasures are people . . .
together.

Realize that it's never too late. Do ordinary things in an ex-
traordinary way. Have health and hope and happiness.
Take the time to wish upon a star.

And don't ever forget, for even a day, how very SPECIAL
you are.

Thank you, Carolyn, for sharing such beautiful thoughts
with all of us. You have offered your friendship to so many
through the website, and now I hope many others will know you
for the special person you are.

Throughout this book (and throughout my life) I've drawn so
much inspiration from the words of others, and when I'm able to, I
like to pass them on. Maybe what works for me will renew someone else's hope or light a little fire of motivation and encouragement inside another person on the journey to good health and
strong self-esteem. Just as we honor heroes for their exploits and res-
cues, so, too, I feel good about focusing attention on those heroes
whose "weapon of choice" is the pen or the computer keyboard!

My friend Barbara popped in to the website one evening

not long ago. After reading a post from a woman looking for help in sticking with a healthy lifestyle, she decided to draw on her own feelings to offer some direction. She forwarded this to me after she posted it, noting that putting her own thoughts into words had helped her, too. (Strange how that works!) I liked what she had to say and wanted to include it here.

> Go back to where the dream began. . . .
>
> It took me a long time to get started again . . . almost a decade since I last lost a lot of weight but didn't manage to keep it off for very long. What got me going again (including a return to a weight-loss support group) and has kept me going (forty-eight pounds so far) is focusing on what I really want . . . what "the dream" is.
>
> I want to like the body in the mirror as much as I love the person inside it. I want to feel a spring in my step when I walk and never get out of breath going up stairs. I want normal blood pressure, not high enough to risk being put on medication. I want to shop for clothes without worrying about elastic waists and gaping buttons. I want to fit into clothes I've been saving to wear again. I want to live a long time and feel good all the way. (And I wouldn't mind fitting into something slinky someday . . . and, oh yes, finding an appreciative boyfriend!)
>
> When I write down those reasons (and more) for myself, I find that the dream is stronger than the urge to keep

eating Chinese stir-fry every day for lunch and dinner (not to mention a pint of ice cream at night!). So far, I haven't struggled much to stay motivated this time around. I've still got lots (forty-plus pounds) to lose, so I imagine those times may come. But I'm convinced that writing down my feelings and reminding myself what's at stake will help. (So will eating food I love from JoAnna's recipes, so I don't feel deprived and stuck eating diet food or midget meals . . .) This is a tough time of year to focus your attention away from food—there's so much around!—but it's way too easy to eat your way from Halloween to New Year's and then comes Valentine's Day candy and Easter chocolate. . . . The food will always be there to tempt us, but the dream is stronger than temptation.

Dream on!

My Healthy Exchanges website isn't the only place on the Web to find support and friendship twenty-four hours a day. Most of the better national weight-loss support groups sponsor such message boards, and a surprising number of individuals who've achieved weight-loss success and wanted to offer help to others have launched their own home pages. Many of the readers who visit Healthy Exchanges also check in with Weight Watchers at weightwatchers.com, a site called Dottisweightlosszone.com, and one I've heard about but haven't visited called 3FatChicks.com that takes a humorous, supportive approach to sharing on the topic.

## A Pearl to Polish

———•———

*Try it tonight—go back to where your dreams began, and write down all the reasons for getting healthy and feeling good about yourself. No dream is too silly or too small to include. Wanting to wear sexy lingerie instead of sturdy underwire support is as legitimate as wanting to bound up a flight of stairs without gasping for breath. Besides, your dreams are yours, in private, so anything goes. Dream big, dream little, then take the steps to make those dreams real.*

# Scaling New Heights

*Supposing you have tried and failed again and again. You may have a fresh start any moment you choose, for this thing we call "failure" is not the falling down, but the staying down.*

—MARY PICKFORD

It's Friday morning, in those wonderful early hours before the sun turns our Iowa cornfields a glorious golden yellow, and I'm about to step onto my scale. There was a time when I feared the scale, when I "dieted" hard the day before and wore the fewest clothes possible. Now it's just a tool I use to record information. More than that, it's become a kind of friend, a partner in my journey to good health and sustained weight loss.

Are you shaking your head in disbelief at that idea? How could a scale, every dieter's harshest critic and fiercest enemy, become an ally? If you'd asked me this about ten years ago, or even twenty, I'd have agreed with you that it was war between me and the scale, and I couldn't imagine a time when I would change my mind about that.

*But I have.*

In those dark days, the scale had the power to hurt me, to shatter my self-esteem, to make me feel worthless and hopeless. Unless it showed me what I wanted to see, I would face the week ahead with dread, and I would use food to comfort the ache inside me. Talk about a vicious cycle.

But because I have learned to accept myself with all my talents and all my flaws, I'm not fighting a war with the scale anymore.

Now I get on the scale once a week, as part of my Reality Check Day, and I look at the number. If I see a small loss of weight from the week before, I smile and say, "Oh, good." If I see that my weight has stayed the same, I silently cheer my victory and think, "Doing fine, JoAnna." And if I see a small weight gain, I say to myself, "What could this mean? Am I practicing what I preach when it comes to moderation? Have I been making good choices when it comes to the restaurants Cliff and I eat in on the road? Did I find enough time to walk or ride my bike this week, or did those long hours in the car make it harder than usual to exercise? Have I been using food to fight fatigue, or simply eating bigger portions than I usually do?"

If the answer to these questions is "No," then I close the little notebook and go about my business. If I've done my best to do what I know works for me, then I don't browbeat myself about what the scale said. (After all, I'm in full-fledged menopause these days. . . .) I know that following my HELP precepts works for me, and I don't need some "quick fix" or "instant weight-loss plan" to lose a couple of unwanted pounds.

But if the answer to any of those questions is "Maybe," or "Yes, I think so," then I feel a kind of quiet gratitude for the scale's reminder. It's like a tap on the shoulder from a friend, a Post-It note on the soul. It is something that tells me that this week I can do better, that I should treat myself with more care and concern for my health. It strengthens my determination to live the lifestyle I've chosen to the fullest extent of my ability. Instead of feeling like a failure because of what the scale says, I accept the information, decide how I am going to cope with it, and *move on* with my life. I'm not going to hide in my room because of a number on the scale. I've got work to do, grandkids to spoil, and a wonderful life to lead, so there is no time for the kind of negative feelings and behavior I used to wallow in a decade ago.

Will I make changes in my life during the upcoming weeks because of what the scale said? Perhaps, but it's because I recognize the need to do something different, to focus better on what I know is best for me. I know that I have the power to change what I do, that I'm the one in charge.

What I've discovered, and a little to my amazement, is that sometimes I do better at living healthy when Cliff and I are on the road than when we're at home. Even when we've got many miles to drive, we have to stop from time to time, so I can get out and get in ten minutes of walking around the car or the truck stop. So on a day when I was nearly certain I'd have to skip my exercise, I get more than I expected—and surprisingly, more than I've gotten on some days at home, when one thing just led to another and suddenly it was bedtime! Cliff does his part, too, parking the car or motor home at the far end of the parking lot, so we get our exercise—and also so people passing by can see that the HELP Wagon has come to town!

For me, it's all about paying attention. I have to recognize that the day doesn't just happen, but that I have some control over how each day of my life unfolds. Sure, there are the unexpected interruptions or emergencies, but I've discovered that having a plan helps me structure my time in a way that gives me confidence that I'll fit everything in that I consider to be important. Some days, when I feel as if I haven't done enough to get my heart rate up, I turn on the radio in the evening, find a song with a good beat, and just start tapping my feet and moving my arms. I've even been known to "dance" in the car when the music is upbeat and I'm taking a break from creating recipes. (I've had a few passing truck drivers honk their horns at my gyrations, but I just smile, knowing they'd feel just as good as I do if they were "dancing in the aisles" like me!

It's easier to blame others when things aren't going well, or focus on all the reasons why you can't do what you say you want to do. It's simpler to say that you're stuck, and then just keep doing what you're doing. What's hard is acknowledging that the power to change is in your hands, and in your heart. I got a note from one reader, Susan, not long ago: "I'm feeling hopeless and powerless over this one issue in my life," she wrote. "No matter how hard I try, I can't stay on an eating plan for more than three days. I'm 35 pounds overweight but it feels like 3,500. It robs me of my joy and I know it affects my walk with the Lord."

She went on to tell me how gung-ho she'd felt after reading my book HELP and buying loads of ingredients for a week of healthy menus. But then, she added, "something got stressful at work, and I went back to the old habit of comfort eating. It's the same pattern over and over, and I don't know how to break it."

I know how she feels, and I bet you do too. Old habits are difficult to change, especially when you understand that Susan's problem is not just with the food she's eating, or with the extra pounds lurking on the scale. It's her feeling that the food is in control, not her.

It's easy to be objective when it's not your life and not your problem being discussed, but let's try to tackle this one together. Susan has a refrigerator full of healthy food, but she isn't eating it. Why? Does eating healthy make her feel deprived? Does she consider the recipes she chose "diet" dishes instead of the kind of comfort food that makes her feel satisfied inside? You can follow an exchange plan diet and choose to eat cottage cheese and carrot sticks, but how will that satisfy you for a lifetime? If you don't enjoy the taste of reduced-calorie bread, then you'll always be longing for a bagel or a piping-hot, fresh-from-the-oven dinner roll. It's the attitude as well as the food that makes you feel powerless, and it's that dieting mentality that defeats so many people who insist they want to change.

I wrote to Susan and suggested she take another look at what she'd prepared in her cooking marathon from my cookbooks, and then I asked her to write down what she was actually eating instead of what she had planned. I also noted that her desire for frequent stimulation and change, illustrated by her "flitting" from one weight-loss program to another, instead of committing to *herself* and her desire to lose weight, conflicted with her feelings of being trapped.

A few weeks later, Susan wrote to me again, and she had

made some important progress. "You were right," she said. "I picked all the plainest recipes and none of your pies when I cooked up a week's worth of meals. I chose tuna instead of salmon, and ground turkey (which I don't really like) instead of lean beef. I told myself that if I ate your macaroni and cheese or a creamy coleslaw, I wouldn't lose weight and then I would have wasted all this time and money. After I read your letter, I decided to go against what my old beliefs told me. I gave it one week, vowing to stick with it, and boy, was I surprised! I had healthy cheesecake for dessert. I made a creamy corn chowder and brought it to work for lunch. And I actually found myself smacking my lips over most of the dinners I made."

She ended by writing that she'd lost two pounds that week, which pleased her no end but, she added, "Learning that I was self-sabotaging was a real eye-opener. I kept looking for a diet that didn't feel like a diet, and all the time I could have been eating foods I liked prepared your way."

Victory! I want you to know that I celebrate your victories as joyfully as I do my own, because it means that you've found your way.

### A Pearl to Polish

*After one of my lectures, a woman came up to me and said, "You just never know what will finally hit home. I think it was in one of your newsletters that I read about a lady who kept putting off making the healthy lifestyle changes she needed to—until someone said, 'A year from now you will* wish that you had started today.' That comment went straight to my heart, and I knew I couldn't wait a moment longer." The woman told me that it had been almost a year to the day that she'd turned over a new leaf, and in addition to losing more than forty pounds, she'd finally been taken off her medication for high blood pressure. That year paid wonderful dividends for her, and I know this next year can do the same for you.

# *If You Always Do What You've Always Done . . .*

---

*We must become the change we want to see.*

—MOHANDAS GANDHI

If you always do what you've always done, you'll always get what you always got. . . ."

Ever heard of a mantra? It's the phrase chanted by people who meditate to help them focus, to get them "into the zone." Well, I heard this one business "mantra" from a friend in publishing whose marketing director wanted the sales force to take a fresh approach with a new line of books. I immediately responded to the message it carries: that if you want something in your life to change, you have to change something in your life. There's usually more than one way to tackle a problem, so you're not wedded to a single approach. But continuing what you're already doing means accepting the same result. Is that what you want? Then keep doing what you're doing. But if you want something else for yourself, then you want and need to make a change.

The question is, *what?* If what you're doing isn't working, it's time to change something. Sometimes even the smallest shift will make a world of difference, but it requires an action from you, and a decision to go where you haven't ever been. (Reminds me of that *Star Trek* slogan, "To boldly go where no man has gone before . . .") Well, I'm not asking you to become a pioneer in space, just a bit of a pioneer in your own territory. Change the terrain; take a fresh look at how you're living your life. I like to think of it as the ripple effect. You know that beautiful series of rings that move ever outward when you toss a pebble into a pool of water? Well, think of all that still water as your life *as it is at this moment.* Now—drop a pebble of a new idea into that unchanging stillness. Maybe you decide to put a temporary rinse in your graying hair to help you look as young as you feel. Suddenly, a more youthful appearance makes you more confident, and you volunteer to lead a committee at your child's school. Or perhaps the subtle change in hair color ignites a desire to go back to the gym and get into better shape. And suppose you do, and then you decide to sign up for your local AIDSWALK and you raise $300 in pledges. What then? Well, you've transformed your life and your world with just a few baby steps!

For years, many of us found ourselves on the dieting treadmill, never actually reaching our destination or goal but covering those same old miles (pounds) again and again. The scenery never changed, the path never varied, and the results, eventually, were always the same. We were still **just dieting.**

One of the main reasons I've been able to jump off that treadmill (and happily, over the past few years, to invite many people to take the leap along with me) is that I was ready to do something different, because I wanted a different result. This time, I wasn't out there searching for the next quick fix or the next magic diet, the one that told me if only I ate special combinations of foods at particular times of day, I'd lose the weight and keep it off forever. This time, I decided I wasn't buying into that philosophy anymore. Just as the mantra says, "If you always do what you've always done, you'll always get what you always got."

But it isn't a matter of changing one thing to escape the dieting mindset. Instead, I had to pay attention to all kinds of bad habits that I and other "weight-loss victims" had pursued for so many years. As I took notes and reflected on what it was time to discard, I developed a little "Still Dieting" quiz that has helped me and others zero in on what was part of the past—and how we wanted to change for the future.

1. If you attend weight-loss support group meetings, do you find that you're skipping meals the day of your weigh-in, then heading home after the meeting to gobble the biggest meal of the week? Do you stop drinking water at least four hours before you step on the scale, because you're afraid of a "water gain"? Do you try on half a dozen outfits to find the lightest-weight clothing that will look decent in public because "every ounce counts"? Are you skipping meetings when you're sure you'll show a gain, promising yourself to starve it off before next week? If so, you are *still just dieting!*

2. Do you work as a short-order cook in your own kitchen? Are you still fixing "real food" for your family while eating skimpy "diet food" yourself, believing that you can force the weight to disappear faster? If so, you are *still just dieting!*

3. Are you so concerned about being "in control" that you write down every morsel *before* it goes into your mouth each day? Are you so obsessed with cutting all fat from your diet that you never allow yourself to eat more than 10 or 15 grams a day? If so, you are *still just dieting!*

4. Are you jumping on the scale several times a day (or even every hour on the hour) instead of only once a week? Do you pack your bathroom scale when you go on vacation, just in case? If so, you are *still just dieting!*

5. Do you tell yourself that it's not worth the effort to dress well or develop a personal style because you're never going to be a model anyway? Are you unwilling to try new activities that could develop into lifelong healthy habits (line dancing, water aerobics) because you don't want to bring attention to yourself? If so, you are *still just dieting!*

Are you ready to throw that "diet monkey" off your back? Are you convinced that doing what you've always done isn't getting you anywhere you want to be? Are you prepared to stop looking for obstacles to making changes in your life and start viewing them as opportunities to grow?

Good! It sounds as if you're determined to see a change in the results you usually get, and that's the first step. Identify what isn't working, then make a change—and keep a close eye out for any signs of "relapse." You see, it's awfully easy to fall back into your old patterns, because you've stuck with them for so many years. But now that you're aiming for a different "end," you require a different "means" to that end.

When I was a professional dieter, I followed a very specific pattern. If I didn't drop ten pounds in a week, I deemed that diet a failure, and I went back to what I'd been doing before. Any weight that had come off went right back on, and the "rebound effect" usually meant that I'd end up even a few pounds heavier than when I'd started.

But changing my goal from losing weight to regaining good health meant breaking my old pattern of one week on, one week off (or one week on, months and months *off*). I knew that one week was only the beginning of a long journey, and I told myself to be patient, to realize that change takes time, and to focus on more than one way of measuring success. By doing that, I finally lost the pounds and inches that had stuck with me for all those "on-off" years. I learned that slow but steady was a pattern that worked—and continues to work.

If you found out from taking the quiz that you were *still just dieting,* good for you. You've got knowledge now that you can use to break the pattern that's trapped you for so long in a no-win situation. This is a quiz you can take again in a couple of months and one I hope that you'll soon be able to "ace" because of the changes you've made in your thinking, your eating, and your behavior. When you get to answer a big "No" to every question, it'll be because you learned to live your new mantra: "If you always do what you've always done, you'll always get what you always got." And I hope you'll have written a new one: "When you decide to stop doing what you've always done, you'll begin to get what you never got!"

### A Pearl to Polish

*Before I came to this point in life, my prayers were selfish ones, asking for what I wanted when I wanted it. Now, my daily prayer is simply, "Please, God, help me help myself, so I may help others for Your honor and glory." And life is much more enjoyable. In the middle of my life, after years of my not "getting it," God gave me the gift of inspiring others to believe in themselves and to change for the better. What gift has He given you, and how are you using it to honor Him?*

# Are You Waiting
# Until You're Thin to Live?

*You can complain because roses have thorns, or you can rejoice because thorns have roses.*

—ZIGGY

*W*hen I was stuck in my old dieter's mind and body, I tended to focus on tomorrow, or next week, or next month, or a few months down the road, when I would finally, at last, be thin! Today was only a means to an end, not something celebrated for itself.

Now that I look back on all those years, I know that I missed out on some very precious time. Oh, I was busy and had a full life, raising kids, working full-time, going to college at night. But too much of the time I spent yo-yo dieting, I also spent waiting to live. Really *live!* Because I figured my real life, the good life, the best part of life, wouldn't begin until I weighed a certain weight, fit into a certain size, looked a certain way in the mirror.

I know I'm not alone in this behavior, either, because I've heard so many people say, "If I can just get through these next three months and get down to X pounds, then I know my life will be better. I'll find a boyfriend. I'll get a better job." I know how they feel, because I spent years feeling exactly like that. But now I know something I didn't know back then. It's something that you may begin to understand as you grow older, although some people I've known never seemed to "get" it: The only life you can count on is the one you are living today. So it's important to make today count, to avoid postponing things that matter to you.

I've heard and read lots of versions of that philosophy, but none that touched me more or put what I'm referring to more accurately—and beautifully, I might add—than Joan Rivers, who was selling some new jewelry pieces on QVC one evening. Inside one of her pendants was a verse that said it all:

> *Yesterday is history.*
> *Tomorrow is a mystery.*
> *Today is a gift from God.*
> *That's why it's called the present.*

What a wonderful sentiment, and how true! But of course we don't need to wear something around our necks to keep this idea in the forefront of our minds. All we each need to ask ourselves is, "Are you waiting until you're thin to live?"

If you're putting off getting your hair styled or having your nails done because your appearance doesn't really matter to you until you're at your goal weight, then the answer is Yes.

If you're avoiding going to parties or business get-togethers because you don't have a thing to wear and you aren't willing to look for attractive clothes in your current size, then the answer is Yes.

If you're postponing a vacation to a dream destination because you can't see yourself enjoying a cruise or a safari or even a weekend at a country inn because of how you look in the mirror, then the answer is Yes.

If you're skipping social events that offer opportunities to meet new people (maybe even a beau!) because you can't imagine anyone being attracted to you until you're at a perfect weight, then the answer is Yes.

Did you answer "yes" to any of the questions I posed? Don't be embarrassed to admit it if you did, because most people I've known who had weight concerns have succumbed to the same kind of delaying tactics. But here's the problem with putting your life on hold until you hit that perfect number and the mirror sings your praises: What if all that life you've been waiting to live turns out to be a letdown or disappointment? What if the social life you've been planning doesn't materialize? What if the only thing that's different is that you've suffered and struggled to diet your way down to a magic number, and you didn't end up "over the rainbow"?

Here's another issue: If you believe you're only lovable and attractive when you reach your goal weight, what happens if you gain a pound or two? Will you hide in your room and wallow in self-disgust until the scale says you're free to go? Do you only love yourself when you're thin, and hate yourself all the rest of the time?

I may be hammering this point a little, but it's such an important one. Happiness can't be tied to a number on the scale or your body's similarity to your favorite TV star's skinny physique. And loving yourself can't be a faucet you turn on and off, where from day to day you can't depend even on yourself for emotional support.

Instead, I want you to recognize that today is a day worth celebrating, and that you don't need any other reason but simply being alive. Let's see: The sun rose, the birds are singing, and you've got all these hours to fill with living. Or the day was gray from the moment you got out of bed, and the rain never stopped from dawn to dusk, but you listened to the rain on the roof and you thought, "What a lovely sound, and how cozy it feels to be inside." Or you had to slosh through puddles to get your errands done and you were soaked to the skin when you got home, but that meant you could strip off your wet clothes and jump right into a hot shower, even if it meant that dinner would be served a little late!

Just a few scenarios for an average day, but each one is filled with seconds and minutes and hours that belong to you. **Now** is your time, and **today** is your best opportunity to practice living fully, to feel alive in every moment of the day.

None of this means that your weight-loss goals don't matter, or that you shouldn't make every effort to work toward your dreams. In fact, the only way you'll ever get to live your dreams is to work on them now, today, this minute, because getting there takes time, usually lots of it. But denying yourself pleasure or friendship or a chance to share delicious food on festive occasions isn't the path to getting there faster. It only leaves you feeling deprived, isolated, and even more susceptible to living only for the future.

Waiting to live also doesn't teach you how to handle what you're hoping to find at the end of your personal rainbow. It's not going to be as perfect as you might imagine, because life never is. But if you've got practice dealing with whatever "reality" tosses your way, heavier or thinner, you're more likely to cope with life's ups and downs when you get to your fantasy destination—and you discover it's just more reality, not the perfect paradise you thought it would be. Just ask your size-4 friend about shopping for clothes—and she'll complain she can't find anything that fits right either! (I know, I know—it's hard to believe. . . .)

Another reason it's important not to live for some distant tomorrow is that you're less likely to take responsibility on a daily basis for getting to that faraway place. With your gaze fixed on the future, it's easier to excuse unconscious snacking or a "just this once" philosophy, because your goal seems so unreal. That's one of the reasons I'm a fan of small, interim goals that keep you grounded in the reality of today. If you're determined to make time for exercise four days a week, and you promise yourself an hour-long phone call to your best friend on Sunday if you meet your goal, you have a very immediate, very specific time frame, and a reward that's close at hand instead of off in the fog of "someday."

So if you've found yourself pinning your gaze on a "future you" instead of the one you're living with right now, why not try to refocus your attention on where you are today, and who you are today? I know that thinking of how you'll feel when you're thinner or healthier is appealing, and I don't want you to deny yourself the pleasure of relishing how reaching your goal will feel. But don't pass up the possibilities of today for the unknown world of tomorrow. Time is precious, whether you've got five pounds, fifty pounds, or more to lose. Live all you can now, live all you can tomorrow, and keep living fully until the last moment of your life. There's no better way to show self-love than making each minute count!

### A Pearl to Polish

*Did you ever notice that when you're truly happy and in your element, time passes so quickly you never have a chance to look at your watch? And when you're feeling miserable, every minute drags? Living in the present, making all you can of every blessed moment, is the best way to enjoy the journey, whatever its length!*

# Asking for Help

*It takes a lot of courage to show your dreams to somebody else.*

—ERMA BOMBECK

$\mathcal{W}$hen I arrived at my desk one morning, I found the following letter right on top of a pile of correspondence: "I have recently discovered your book *HELP*, and I must say that you could not have named it more appropriately. I have been asking God for help, and He saw fit to remind me that help usually comes in the form of action. Thank you so much for sharing your knowledge on living a healthier lifestyle. You have given me hope for the first time in years."

Talk about starting your day with a boost!

This particular note, from a lady in Texas, touched my heart very deeply. From the moment I began working on *HELP* all those years ago, I hoped it would help me fulfill what I believed was my own ministry and mission from the Lord: to share my ideas, inspiration, and encouragement with others, to help them achieve what I had achieved with the grace of God, a life of better health after a lifetime of struggling with negative feelings and behaviors.

There are a very few among us who can reach great goals without the help of others, and without the inspiration that comes from a belief in a higher power. And yet, again and again, I hear from people who say rather apologetically, "Well, I really need some group support to keep motivated," or "I know I should be able to follow your program by reading the book, but I felt confused and didn't know where to turn."

No matter what you might read in the press, nobody does it all alone. Asking for help, and accepting help from others, is the secret weapon of all successful people. And it makes sense, doesn't it? Isolation is the toughest place from which to make life changes, because you have no one to turn to when you're feeling frustrated, and no one to rely on when the going gets tough. I've been so pleased to see people acting as a support group for each other using the Healthy Exchanges website, and I know that the Web features dozens of helpful sites where people working on weight loss and other lifestyle changes can offer advice, share information, and "pat each other on the back," in a manner of speaking!

When you've got an aching tooth, you think nothing of phoning the dentist for an appointment, and no one would expect you to sew up your own wound after a kitchen accident, right? But still you hear people say, "Oh, I'd rather do it myself," as if that makes them better people than those who join groups, participate in online chats, and seek the advice of friends and family.

Well, I'm a staunch believer in asking for help (whether you ultimately take the advice you're given or not!). And I've also learned along the way to be gracious when people offer suggestions, even if I feel I'm doing just fine already. I'm not so perfect that I think I know everything there is to know about living healthy. I talk with dietitians and doctors and fitness specialists to get the benefit of their wisdom, and I incorporate what I learn and what I read into my lectures and newsletter. After all, think how much we could all learn if thousands focused on the same problem instead of just a few. Even when I think I've figured out a dozen great variations on a popular recipe, I'm thrilled when someone writes to me with a new version or a family-pleasing change.

The same is true when you're tackling the journey of living healthy in the real world. Sure, there is an abundance of information to wade through, so you don't have to take or accept it all. But keeping an open mind is vital for anyone who doesn't want to remain mired in the past, revisiting old failures and letting history repeat itself. A famous philosopher, George Santayana, once wrote, "Those who cannot remember the past are condemned to repeat it."

But how do we learn from history, and how do we change the future so it's not more of the same? I think that a great start is asking for help, looking for fresh ideas that offer new opportunities for growth.

Let's say that you've signed up at your local gym to get in some exercise. It's expensive, and not very convenient, but you figure it's the best way to get and stay motivated. The only thing is, last year you joined and then never seemed to get there more than once a week. Is it a good way to spend your hard-earned money? Is it working for you, or do you need help?

Why not make a list of options, so on those days and weeks when getting to the gym seems an impossibility, you can still get your lungs pumping in some other way? Let's start with something simple: walking. Do you live in a neighborhood where it's safe to walk alone in the early morning or at night? Would it be safer if you had a walking partner? Who else could you ask to join you for a twice-weekly morning walk before you head off to work?

Maybe, though, you're worried about not having enough time to spend with your kids, and making time for exercise feels like time stolen away from them. One of my readers told me she and her teenage daughter schedule a walk together after dinner several nights a week. "We cheerfully leave the dishes on the table—not even in the sink!—and we head out for a good thirty to forty-five minutes. It's been some of the best time together we've ever had, and it's been amazing how much closer it's made us feel. Not only that, but I feel as if I really know how her life is going, and I think she feels that she can share her feelings with me more than she ever did before."

That's how Sally solved her exercise scheduling challenge, but maybe you're single and a city dweller who doesn't feel safe heading out after dark, and you leave for work too early in the morning to plan much of a workout then. That's your starting point, but don't give up just yet. Do you have a secret yen to learn country line dancing, or have you dreamed of gliding around a ballroom in a graceful waltz? Most major cities offer a variety of dance class options, and you may also find some as part of your local high school's adult education program. Dancing has always been one of my favorite exercises, and you can work up quite a sweat even doing the fox-trot!

One of the biggest complaints I hear about exercising is that people get bored, so I was delighted to hear the solution one group of friends tried recently. "We've all got a few exercise videos, but most of us had grown tired of them. So we decided to have a grab-bag exchange and trade once a month. Each of us wraps up one of our favorites in pretty gift paper and brings it to an informal brunch at one of our houses. As we're ready to leave, each of us 'gets a gift' at the door and goes home with a new fitness workout to try. Since we never know what we're going to get, it's fun—and motivating!"

I've discovered that this kind of help is easy to ask for. What's harder is the kind of emotional support that keeps us focused on the road to better health. I've talked with and written to many people who are going through difficult and even tragic times. While I've certainly encouraged them in their efforts to eat well and get some exercise, I know that they may need more than I can give them. One mother had lost her teenage son in a terrible car accident; another was caring for aging parents who both had Alzheimer's; and many others were coping with illness themselves. There are wonderful support groups for parents who've lost children, for cardiac and cancer patients, and still others that provide respite care for exhausted caregivers. *Please don't try to go it alone.* Often, a clergyperson can provide enormous comfort in difficult times, but sometimes what you really need is to talk and share with others in the same boat. If you can't find such a group close to home, or you're in a rural area, perhaps you'll find kindred spirits online, or even a pen pal (yes, people are still writing letters even now that the millennium has rolled around!) through an organization. Sometimes, strangers can provide more comfort than close friends or relatives, because you don't feel you have to be brave for them. You can be angry, bitter, scared, and honest—and you can get the help you really need.

Sometimes, of course, the only help many of us need is knowing that we are not alone, that the Lord is with us every day and through the darkest nights. I have always taken tremendous comfort in that knowledge, and in my faith in God. For some who may not have a close connection with a church or synagogue, or for those who have lost touch with a faith that once provided guidance, perhaps it is time to find your courage, to reach out and seek this kind of connection. And if you've been a regular attendee at services but have never sought out your minister for a private conversation, maybe it's a good time to do so. There may be many people in your town or congregation who long to make connections with others, who need support in a life struggle but don't know how to begin. Perhaps you will, by reaching out and asking for help, transform not only your own life but that of others. It's amazing how much light one small candle can give in a pitch-dark room, and how warm the glow of faith can grow from that first spark.

### A Pearl to Polish

*Just as joy shared is multiplied, so too is the potential for change and growth when you dare to invite someone else to share your journey on the path to healthy living. If you've been struggling in isolation for a while now, why not give someone the chance to offer advice to help you over a rough spot? (The secret, of course, is that you don't have to take the advice, but opening a dialogue with a friend or family member opens a way for both of you to take more steps in the direction of your goal to live better and feel better.)*

# Where Can I Cash My Reality Check?

*Okay, who stopped the payment on my reality check?*
—BUMPER STICKER

$O$ne of my favorite slogans, one I chose for my business (and myself) a long time ago, is "Living Healthy in the Real World." I have dreams and fantasies, just as we all do, but the place I hang my hat is *real*. The person I see in my mirror is a real, middle-aged grandmother, not some overly made-up and perfectly slimmed-down celebrity. I do the best I can with what I've got, but I recognize that there are limits to what even a good hairdresser, well-made clothing, and an optimistic attitude can accomplish. Whether I'm wearing silk or denim, whether I'm made up for a television appearance (which requires loads more makeup than I would ever wear on the street!) or I'm riding my bike around DeWitt in the peaceful hours just after dawn without a drop of foundation on my cheeks—I'm the same, real person inside, and I'm blessed to know that.

But reality is not always an easy place to live.

It's full of mirrors that encourage us to criticize our bodies. It's peopled with so-called "friends" and even relatives who believe that pointing out our shortcomings is the only way to "help" us change. They may say, "Get real"; but urging us to give up favorite foods, dress more conservatively, act our age, or accept our failings isn't doing us a favor at all.

I've heard some people say that you create your own reality, and that's an interesting philosophy, but I think what you truly create is how you handle the reality you face. To help myself do it better, I came up with the concept of Reality Check Day, a system that has helped me lose more than 130 pounds and keep it off for nearly ten years now.

Most people with a weight problem become obsessed about it, looking for constant evidence that whatever they're "doing"— a high-protein diet, a new exercise class, even a cellulite-reducing cream they're spreading on their thighs—is working. So they jump on the scale every hour on the hour, and if they don't see some downward movement, they give up.

Now, I'm not saying that you don't need to check on your progress from time to time while you're working on lifestyle changes, but since the goal is "reality," not the fantasy of instant gratification, you want a sensible and reasonable approach to doing just that.

Here's a good analogy of what I mean: When you're driving cross-country from San Francisco to Washington, D.C., you don't check the map every five minutes or every mile marker. (I hope you don't, anyway, or you'd never get there!) Instead, you check it at reasonable intervals: if the entire trip will take a week, you may check it once a day. You choose a few intervals to double-check that you're on the right track, and the rest of the time you concentrate on the road and the view. But your weight-loss journey and the trip to better health will take months, maybe years. That's okay. Remember—it's not only the destination but the journey that matters in life!

I think you'll find that the concept of Reality Check Day works. To help you declare your independence from the bondage of "just dieting" instead of living healthy in the real world, I suggest you monitor your progress *no more than once a week.* This means no more sneaking over to your scale in the middle of the night to see if you're being "good." Can you do that? Or does the prospect of cutting those apron strings make you incredibly nervous?

I know that it might, but here's why it's important to keep the *real* goal in mind: Linking your self-esteem and your commitment to your health to something as unreliable (yes, unreliable!) as your bathroom scale is downright dangerous. Success is motivating, absolutely, but without hard evidence that your healthy eating and your steady exercising are making a measurable difference you may decide to give up—and that's no good.

I've often talked about the power of faith and how important it is to believe in yourself and what you're doing to become healthier. Well, I'm convinced that Reality Check Day empowers you by removing the temptation to judge yourself on a daily basis. Instead, you look at the numbers one day a week—and the rest of the time, you focus on living your life, instead of searching for the flaws in you or your diet. It's simple, and it's powerful—and take it from me, it works!

So, how to begin? I suggest doing your Reality Check on the same day each week, and at the same time of day if you can. Wear the same or similar clothes and take your measurements at the same places on your body, aiming for accuracy and consistency. If losing weight is your goal, as it was mine, start by climbing on the scale for a private weigh-in. I created a chart to keep track of the numbers, and it's also fun to draw a little graph showing your progress along the way.

Then get out your trusty tape measure and measure what I call the "weight-loss checkpoints," all those places that slim down and tighten up over time as you eat healthy and exercise moderately: the neck, chest, waist, hips, upper arms, upper thighs, and calves.

Why measure yourself if you're not intending to compete in bodybuilding competitions or planning to expose your physique in public? Simply put, progress doesn't always show up on the scale, but your body is slowly and wonderfully transforming itself into a more efficient machine. Because exercising can help you replace fat with muscle, and because muscle actually weighs more than fat, you might not see a weight loss for a week or even two. But your legs may be growing stronger and your hips slimming down, whether you notice it or not!

(Don't forget, by the way, that when you're adding up the inches lost, you include both arms and both legs!)

The other part of Reality Check Day is writing down everything you eat, and measuring carefully. Do it once a week, and the rest of the time, you can feel confident that three ounces of meat hasn't grown to six ounces, or that you're not eating out of control. By doing this, you stay aware of what you consume in an average day, and it helps keep you on track. When I first began, it took me about two months to get to the point of doing it this way. It takes some people longer before they choose to give up keeping a daily record, and that's fine. It's all part of "lightening up" on yourself so that your body will "lighten up" on you. Otherwise, it becomes too easy to become obsessed about being perfect, about eating exactly five bread servings or five protein servings, so that all you do all day is think of food. (On the other hand, if keeping a food journal is a way that helps you in your effort to live healthy, I'm not going to discourage you from using whatever tools are available. It's *your* choice—but I want you to know that you have one!)

Many long-term dieters may hesitate to go with my once-a-week suggestion, concerned that they'll forget what they've eaten, or go overboard if they fail to write down every single morsel of food. But once you get in tune with your body and build confidence in your ability to eat healthily, you'll find that this is a liberating approach that may transform the way you relate to food.

People ask if I still continue with Reality Check Day, all these years later, and my answer is a resounding "Yes!" Since I'm sometimes on the road for more than a week, I don't do it every week, but I *do* do it. I keep a scale in my dressing room, and a little notebook with my measurements. I'm still accountable to myself (the only person who needs to know these numbers!) and I'm still living in the real world, keeping in touch with what the facts are, not with what I want the facts to be.

A friend once told me that her support group leader said she wished she could weigh her members only once a month, because women's bodies fluctuate so much, the scale often didn't show what was really happening. I mention that only to remind you that the scale is just one measure of what is changing in your life with each week that you commit to a healthy lifestyle. Yes, sometimes you'll see weight loss and other times you'll notice that your clothes fit you better. Sometimes you'll catch a glimpse of yourself in a store window and say, "You know, I look *good*." And often the only change that is occurring is occurring inside you—in the strengthening of your commitment to change, in your confidence that you can reach your goals, in your lightening up on yourself *inside* as you begin to on the outside.

A reality check is a promise you make to yourself, that you are willing and brave enough to be aware of what you're eating or of whether you're making time to walk. It's saying, "My life is going to be lived positively from now on." With so much self-knowledge, you will feel yourself evolving, being transformed, and getting in touch with your true self.

So even if you'll always be a size larger on the bottom as I am, or even if your officemates suggest this new diet or that new appetite suppressant, why not just smile and say, "I'm living in the real world now. And from where I stand, it looks beautiful!"

### A Pearl to Polish

*You don't need a pair of rose-colored glasses to get through life with a positive attitude. But you do need a willingness to gaze* clear-eyed into the mirror and recognize that what is reflected isn't the entire picture of who you are. What is essential is the heart and soul of a person; that's what is most real, most true, and it's how God and small children see us. Practice just for today seeing yourself and others with innocence and kindness. Make your strongest reality a spiritual one.

# Getting Up
# with the Cows

---

*Since the early bird catches the worm, it's a good idea to begin
your day as soon as you can—unless, of course, you happen to
be a worm.*

—EDWIN BLISS, AUTHOR

*R*emember that old song from
the sixties "Time Is on My Side"? We sang along to it when the
Rolling Stones drove home the message, but deep down, I think
most of us never really believed it. Or, if we believed it back then
when life seemed much less complicated, it's definitely harder to
believe it now!

I'm the mother of three, the grandmother of five. I've got a
husband to take care of and a business we run together. I do my
own laundry and most of my own cleaning up. I create dozens of
recipes a week, write my books and my newsletter, draft public-
ity releases, appear on radio and television programs at all hours

of the day and evening. When we used to cater Healthy Exchanges meals as part of a presentation, I served the pies or spooned up the mashed potatoes if help was needed.

To put it simply, I'm busy. But I'm not unique in having a very full life; I know that. What I want to share with you are some of the ways I keep myself from going crazy with all that I have to do, and all that I *want* to do.

First and maybe foremost, I get up with the cows. I think this habit began when I was a young mother getting up early to care for my children. But as my sons and daughter grew up and left home, I kept it going. (I'd pretty much reset my body clock after so much time.) And those minutes and hours before the rest of the world begins humming have become more important to me over the years.

I feel a jumble of emotions as I get out of bed—a sense of expectancy and curiosity about what's to come, a determination to fill the day with good and satisfying work, and a feeling of being at peace with the world. As I shower and dress, I ask myself, What will the new day hold? What hopes and dreams will today make possible, and what exciting results will the hard work of recent weeks and months produce?

But before I begin the practical activities that fill my early hours, I pause and take time to commune with God. I know how much of my strength comes from reaching out to Him, and I feel grateful for an unrushed opportunity to express gratitude for the gift of this new day. In those private moments, in that silent house, I think about the many blessings I have been given and how I have tried to use them for His glory and for good. It's in those peaceful minutes, in that stillness, that I discover new purpose and begin to understand how to achieve what He has planned for me.

Living in a world full of interruptions and distractions, it's not easy to find precious time to reflect on your life and refresh your soul. But nothing I do or have ever done is as vital to my happiness and my success as a human being than taking a few minutes each morning to make a spiritual connection. I keep it private, I keep it simple, and I keep it wherever I happen to find myself that morning. I like to think of this brief interlude as my soul's multivitamin, my spirit's Daily Requirement, and I know my life would be less without it.

Once I've taken care of heart and soul in that way, I tackle the other needs of the heart, the lungs, the muscles, and so on. I've always preferred to exercise in the morning, whether I'm striding along the highway in the warm summer months or pounding the rug from room to room as I "walk my house" because it's just too cold outside! I bend and stretch, taking inventory of how a night's rest has refreshed my body (or not), and paying attention to what my physical self is telling me. I remember how awful it felt to wake up creaky, exhausted, in pain from a dozen big and little aches caused by being seriously overweight. My memory may occasionally be fuzzy about some things, but that's a sensation I won't ever forget—and one I don't want to repeat if I can help it!

I've become very attached to feeling good in my body, and I'm willing to keep doing what it takes to keep it in shape for the demands of my daily life. It's all part of my philosophy of moderation in all things. I don't need a strenuous, sweaty workout every morning and night to attain my fitness goals, and I don't aspire to be an Olympic marathon runner (not even in my dreams!).

What I want is a healthy heart, muscles that are strong enough to lift my grandbabies, a back that will support me when I work for hours at my stove testing recipes or at my computer writing my newsletter. I need stamina, endurance to get me through very full days of work and family responsibilities. So walking, riding my bike, and dancing are usually my chosen forms of exercise, and making the commitment to keep my body moving on a daily basis has been an important element in sustaining my 130-pound weight loss of ten years ago.

I also love the early morning because my mind is very clear and open, not yet cluttered with all the demands of the workday. It's a great time to select a theme for my editor's corner, which we now call "Straight From the Heart." It's a terrific time to think of new ideas for cookbooklets for the next five years. It's a wonderful time to read through letters that ask me to make over recipes in my Healthy Exchanges way—and it's a perfect time to figure out on paper just how I might do it!

Before I know it, the sun is up, the house is stirring, cars and trucks begin heading up and down the highway, and the day is well under way. My "getting up with the cows" time is over for today, but I'm satisfied with all I managed to accomplish. I'm ready to tackle the rest of the day with renewed energy, and I've got a to-do list with all my priorities clear. Instead of waking up late and heading fuzzy-brained into phone-ringing chaos, I'm warmed up (as athletes must be before they race) and I'm ready to go.

Now, what can you do to make yourself ready to run the race of *your* life? Maybe you've never been an early riser, and so the theme of this chapter is more horrifying than inspiring. Maybe you've been getting up early for years with your kids, and now that they're in college, you're reveling in a chance to sleep a little later!

Well, getting up with the cows is not a requirement for success in life, I promise you, though it has been very good for me. But carving out time to connect with your spiritual needs and your heart's true desires is a worthwhile goal for everyone. Maybe your golden hours are after midnight, when your family has gone to bed and you've just turned off the news. Or perhaps your most peaceful time is a precious lunchtime break that you spend walking in the park near your office.

What I am suggesting is that you take what may be an informal, occasional, incidental part of your life and make a daily commitment to it. (If that's not possible right now, begin with a few times a week.) By setting aside some regular time for thinking, breathing, dreaming, praying, and reflecting, I believe you will effect a quiet but significant transformation in your life.

It may mean getting up a half hour earlier, or arranging for car-pooling help a day or two a week. It may produce feelings of guilt at first, since you're used to putting everyone else's needs before your own. And it may actually be more frustrating than productive at first because it takes time to trust the process of what you're trying to do. It's much the same with the practice of formal meditation: at first, you don't know what you're supposed to be thinking about, but you're pretty sure you're doing it wrong. Or you can't see any immediate results, and you're used to striving for what you can see and touch and feel.

But this is a practice that gets better, the longer and more fully you do it. Just keep it simple, take notes if it feels right to you, and pay attention to the little "pokes" and "prods" you get from your mind and heart while you're making contact with yourself.

### A Pearl to Polish

*Sometimes the truest parts of you emerge when it feels most safe, and this time you're setting aside for reflection will call forth what is deepest and perhaps unrevealed. Open your mind, open your heart, open your eyes, and welcome the "inside" parts of you into the world. Trust what your instincts tell you in the clearheaded, quiet times, and use what you're discovering about yourself to grow.*

# Finding the Courage to Face Your Fears

*You gain strength, courage, and confidence by every experience
in which you really stop to look fear in the face. . . . You must
do the thing you think you cannot do.*

—ELEANOR ROOSEVELT

$\mathcal{W}$e all know what it's like to feel
afraid—of meeting someone new, confronting a challenge at
work, or maybe just coming to terms with a few gray hairs. But
even though such fears are universal, we often try to disguise the
fact that we're shaking in our shoes. After all, if people know
we're scared or feeling insecure, they'll take advantage of us,
right?

Have you ever watched very young children encounter the
world with expressions of pure joy and astonishment? Fear isn't
yet in their vocabulary, and each new experience inspires wonder,
not concern. In fact, parents have to *teach* children to be a little

afraid in order to ensure their safety—telling them Don't touch the stove, Stay out of the street, Don't talk to strangers, and so on.

But as adults, we find that too often fear paralyzes us and keeps us from trying something new or changing what's not working in our lives. Finding the strength to face that fear and conquer it isn't easy, but sometimes it's our only hope for a better, happier, healthier life.

Not long ago, I met Evelyn, a recent widow whose children were grown and who had decided to go back to work. She'd gotten married young and had never finished college. The only jobs she'd ever held were hourly sales positions, but the store where she'd worked had closed long ago. She had come to hear me speak about living a healthier life, but as she waited in line to have a book autographed, she was thinking about more than just losing a few pounds. We began chatting as I signed her book, and after a few minutes, she said, "I know that getting back in shape will give me more confidence, and maybe make me look and feel a little younger. But I'm so afraid no one will want to hire a woman of my age, someone who hasn't typed a letter since high school. I can balance a checkbook perfectly, and I've always been good with figures, but when I watch my grandkids working on the computer, I'm just overcome with doubt."

Does Evelyn's story sound familiar? I bet there are many of you in your fifties and beyond who are feeling left behind by this confusing new world of computers and chat rooms, e-mail and Web sites. Not knowing how to do what "everyone else" seems to can quickly shatter your confidence. You could accept the situation, keep doing what you've always done, and if you share

Evelyn's fears, eventually settle for a job that may be poorly paid and unsatisfying.

But *you have a choice.* You can admit your ignorance—and you can do something about it. Stop by your local library or bookstore and pick up a copy of one of those "Dummies" or "Idiot's" books about the Internet; sign up for an adult education class at the high school and find out that a mouse is nothing to be afraid of; ask your favorite grandchild to teach you what he's doing with all those colorful screens.

Above all, don't let a false pride or fear of embarrassment keep you from learning something *new.* Education should be a lifelong journey, but too often adults expend all their energy raising their families, working long hours, and squeezing in a little leisure activity. Many of these hardworking people think they're too old to pick up new skills or learn a language, so they won't even try.

Evelyn is coping with more than just a fear of the job market. She's still grieving for the husband who shared her life for nearly thirty-five years. She's facing the world on her own after decades of seeing herself as primarily wife and mother; she needs a fresh purpose in her life after years of caring for her children and doing volunteer work. I found the perfect quote for her scribbled in one of my notebooks: "The cure for sorrow is to learn something new." And I'm glad to report that Evelyn found the courage to face her fears, and she's dared to venture somewhere she'd never imagined going. She's now back in college part-time, working in the financial aid office, and using a computer every day in her accounting classes.

So think about it: What fear is holding you back? What *don't* you do because it makes you uncomfortable? Did you turn down a chance to go canoeing with your kids last summer because you've never been a very good swimmer? Did you send your regrets when you were asked to give a talk at the library about your trip to Alaska because speaking in public makes you too nervous? Are you still wearing that same baggy black dress to parties, even though you've recently lost twenty pounds and would look better in something more colorful and fitted?

Fear is a kind of shadow emotion. If we don't talk about it, if we hide our feelings from even those closest to us, if we come up with perfectly acceptable alibis for why we're not participating fully in life, we think we've won, or at least postponed the confrontation. But it's ourselves we're hiding from, and our fears that we cannot truly escape.

Eleanor Roosevelt was a shy young woman who married a man she admired, a man whose destiny was politics and a prominent role on the world stage. When polio made it impossible for Franklin Delano Roosevelt to travel around the country and share his message, Mrs. Roosevelt had to take his place. An accident of fate forced her into the public eye, and though she found it extraordinarily difficult at first, what she most feared—meeting strangers and speaking to large groups—transformed her. She grew into her new job and found her own remarkable voice, becoming an inspiration to all those who heard her.

Sometimes, our fears tell us what we need to do, even if we're unaware that anything is wrong. When my daughter, Becky, was pregnant with her first child, I did my best to stay in touch while I carried on with my extremely busy schedule. I was touring for my books, speaking to groups around the country, doing interviews, and visiting bookstores, all the while supervising dozens of employees and running a business that included a restaurant and gift shop. But when Becky needed me and I desperately wanted to go to her, I couldn't. I had so many commitments, I couldn't be there for my only daughter. It was a real shock to the system, a true eye-opener that I couldn't ignore. Cliff and I had built our business into something to be proud of, but instead of *our* running the business, *it* was running our lives. I felt a combination of fear and relief when I made the difficult decision to step back, to do *less* instead of more, as I always had tried to do. I knew some people might criticize my decision, but at least I wasn't afraid of that. The very real fear that I was losing control of my life was a catalyst to change it. By facing my fear and what it represented, I won my freedom.

You can, too!

Tonight, when the dinner dishes are done, and you can grab a few minutes of quiet time, sit down with a pad and a pen. Then ask yourself: What am I most afraid of? How do I feel "stuck"? What would I change if I could?

Be as honest as you can, and remember that "confessing" the truth to yourself can be difficult, even upsetting. Sometimes, living in denial is simply easier than coming to terms with what isn't working in your life. But once you do, you've got the beginnings of a plan.

Pick one thing from your list, and then write down up to five ways you could start to face that fear. Break down each way into a few steps, and decide what you will do tomorrow. Yes, *tomorrow.* Don't put it off, or you'll succeed in talking yourself out of doing it.

### A Pearl to Polish

*Fear can be very persuasive, but you have more strength than you know. Think of a time when you did something diffi-cult—passed your driving test, learned to touch-type, asked your boss for a raise. You did it before, and you can do it now.*

# You Can't Please Everyone . . .

*Only I can change my life. No one can do it for me.*

—CAROL BURNETT

$\mathcal{W}$hen summer is in full swing out here in the heartland, I find myself singing the words to Ricky Nelson's song "Garden Party" almost every day. Maybe my age is showing, but Ricky will always be a special "heartthrob" of my youth. What was not to love? He was cute, could sing great, and got along with his parents! I used to watch him all the time on *Ozzie and Harriet,* and I especially loved the shows where he got to sing. I still join in whenever I hear one of his songs on the radio, and it was never more true than the last time I heard that wonderful voice singing "Garden Party." For some reason, I found myself listening to his words instead of his voice. Those words reached out and touched my soul in a totally unexpected way, and I was amazed to discover that Ricky's message was even better and more powerful than his beautiful music!

When the last line of the song had finally faded away, I knew that "Garden Party" should be proclaimed the "Theme Song" for *anyone* and *everyone* trying to make healthy living choices that are right for each of us. It's exactly right for all of us endeavoring every day to do the best we can . . . *the best we can*. If you're not familiar with the words to this Ricky Nelson classic, I'll share the theme that I believe truly says it all: *You can't please everyone, so you've got to please yourself.*

These could be the most important ten words you'll ever take to heart, so say them aloud, along with me, right now: *You can't please everyone, so you've got to please yourself.* Now, repeat this sentence to yourself at least once a day until it becomes part of your permanent "healthy thoughts memory bank." I'm not encouraging you to be selfish when I suggest you commit to this belief, and certainly not urging you to think, "Me first at all costs." But I do consider it a terrific confirmation, putting into words that you're dedicating yourself to doing what's best for you.

Have you noticed that not everyone is thrilled when you begin making healthier lifestyle choices? Some people may actually resent the fact that you have committed the time and effort to losing weight, lowering your cholesterol, or stabilizing your blood sugar. The reasons may vary from plain old jealousy to annoyance that their *old* daily habits may be compromised by your *new* ones.

So what do you do if you can't please everyone? Just remember Ricky's words: "You can't please everyone, so you've got to please yourself."

Are you willing to toss your healthy lifestyle choices overboard just because some friends, family members, or co-workers turn green with envy because "you're really doing it" this time? I hope not! What if one of these concerned friends says to you, "I see you've lost some weight. How long do you think you'll keep it off this time?" You could respond with anger at the implied message that your weight loss won't last, that you'll soon backslide and maybe even end up heavier than you were when you began. You could react defensively and tentatively, saying, "Well, umm, I'm not—um, I don't—" showing this person just how much power she has over your emotions. Instead, why not smile and politely say, "I'm so glad you noticed. I feel so much better. Excuse me, I see someone I promised to visit with tonight." Why let that person's resentment of your accomplishments turn what you should rightly feel proud of into a mass of self-doubt? Remember, *you can't please everyone, so you've got to please yourself.*

I've gotten letters from people with just this kind of "relationship" problem. One woman wrote that her best girlfriend was upset that she couldn't count on her anymore to split a large pizza topped with everything. She didn't want to give up the friendship, but there had to be a better compromise than chowing down on half a pizza! I suggested that they order a smaller pizza, topped half with her favorite veggies, and the other half with her friend's favorite toppings. She could have one or two slices, leave the rest for her friend, and not make an issue of it. That way, she's not trying to become a zealot or change the way the world eats, but she's also not becoming a pushover for someone else's less-than-healthy choices. Remember, *you can't please everyone, so you've got to please yourself.*

But what if your kids have their hearts set on a fast-food celebration of the soccer team's victory, and you'd have more to choose from at another kind of restaurant? The choice is yours, but knowing how many alternative choices to high-fat burgers and chicken nuggets are now available, I think you can still please your kids without betraying yourself. A small hamburger and a garden salad with lite dressing will nourish you while not denying them a special splurge. I offer this example to show that it doesn't have to be about one person "giving in" while the rest get what they want. But I also believe that it's up to you to speak up when the gang is deciding where to head after a game or party, and if you'd prefer an Italian restaurant over a barbecue joint, *say so!* Don't expect people to be mind readers or "sacrifice" what they want because they know you're trying to eat healthier meals—participate in the decision making and you won't feel as if your wishes don't matter.

The bottom line in making healthy living choices is assessing what's appropriate for you, and then doing it. If you don't make time for your daily walks, then you can't count on anyone else doing it for you. If you don't make preparing healthy meals a priority, then they won't appear by magic in your freezer or fridge (unless you've got some great elves I don't know about!). And if you don't value yourself enough to pat yourself on the back when you make good decisions, you can't depend on someone else's noticing and congratulating you.

There was a bestselling business book some years ago that

took the point of view that you had to put yourself first or you'd never get ahead, that it was every man for himself when it came to survival in the dog-eat-dog, cutthroat business world. That seems to me a kind of extreme version of what I'm talking about here.

But most of us are bombarded daily with the opinions and attitudes of others, and we have to decide how we are going to cope with and handle them. When you receive a promotion at work, some colleagues are genuinely thrilled for you, while others may undercut your achievements and downplay your abilities. Do you reject the opportunity for higher pay and more responsibility so you can keep peace in the typing pool, or do you acknowledge what is usually true: *You can't please everyone, so you've got to please yourself.*

Maybe your mother-in-law doesn't like the car you drive or feels that the living room rug you've chosen is too expensive. Do you return the car keys to the dealer and drive a car someone else prefers instead of sticking with your own choice? Do you deny yourself something beautiful you and your spouse have decided you can afford in order to pour oil on troubled waters, or do you stick to your guns? *You can't please everyone, so you've got to please yourself.*

Making healthy living choices requires the same kind of self-respect. Why not start today by pleasing yourself and begin working toward a small goal that *you* set for *yourself?* Let it be a private matter, unless you choose to share it with someone else. Your progress toward that goal can be something you share with others, or you can decide to keep it private for a while. (Not everyone wants to call Mom after each weekly weigh-in!)

The important thing is making a commitment to doing what you believe is right for you. You may run into obstacles to your goal on a regular basis, and each time you'll need to decide how to handle them. Some days, your goal of eating healthy will seem simple, while on other days, you'll find yourself struggling to make the best choices. Some weeks you'll make time for exercise every single day, and some weeks you may not.

No matter the speed of your progress, you know in your heart and soul that your efforts will pay off. You'll reach your goal, you'll set new ones, and you'll keep trying to do the best you can. But whether there's snow on the ground or an abundance of flowers outside your window, remember the follow-up message of Ricky Nelson's "Garden Party." *In the end, if you don't please yourself, you really can't please anyone else.*

### A Pearl to Polish

*Just for today, do something to please yourself without wondering how someone else will react. Rearrange the furniture in your den; put fresh flowers in a little vase by the bathroom sink; stir your coffee with a cinnamon stick just for fun; put on an outfit you love that your mother or grandmother might suggest is "too young" for you. Since every day is a new beginning, you get to choose how old you feel, and today you're younger than springtime, as the song goes!*

# Letting Go

*Believe in yourself! Have faith in your abilities! Without a humble but reasonable confidence in your own powers, you cannot be successful or happy.*

—DR. NORMAN VINCENT PEALE

Think back to when you were a little child and you longed for independence, to experience the whole wide world on your own. Up to that point, you'd always held tight to your mom or dad's hand, but at that moment, the desire to roam free became stronger than your need for the kind of security that comes from hanging on to what you already know.

Something similar occurs when you decide to follow a healthy lifestyle after years of struggle. You've chosen to lose weight once and for all, you're ready to stick with good habits, you're determined to make today count—and you're finally ready to let go.

Sometimes we have to make a real point of letting go before

we can move forward. It's not enough to say we've changed; we need to act on that decision in a way that breaks with the past and frees us to live unencumbered in the present. It's a kind of spring cleaning for the soul, but you don't have to wait for March or April to get started. Any time of year is a good time to do it, and you'll be astonished how light a little letting go will make you feel.

I started letting go with some obvious things, like deciding I could still live happily ever after without gorging on cake donuts or bingeing on hot fudge sundaes. But traveling along the path to good health meant much more than simply eliminating some unhealthy splurges that had always left me feeling bad.

Something I had to let go of before I really began living healthy was closets full of clothes. I had four full closets packed so tight I could not get another thing into them! The garments inside ranged in size from 8s and 10s to size 28s that had once been way too tight for me. Why did I have so many clothes to deal with? Well, I have always loved designing, and before I became so involved with recipe creation and writing, I used to do the same kind of thing with fabric and fashion. It wasn't uncommon for me to wake up at 5 A.M., sew a new outfit, and wear it to work that very day! But the real reason for my abundance of dresses, skirts, blouses, and so on was more complicated. Because I was always on some new diet, I couldn't be sure what size I'd be wearing from one month to another. If the latest starvation plan was working, then I'd fit into some size 16s or 18s, but I just couldn't force myself to weed out the larger sizes. I didn't have any confidence that I'd be staying where I was, and I just knew that before long I'd need those bigger clothes again. As for those size 8s and 10s that I'd worn almost thirty years ago, well, hope springs eternal in the dieter's heart, and I still believed that someday I might fit into them again. (Never mind that they'd be so far out of style I wouldn't be caught dead wearing them, even if by some miracle I could actually zip them up!)

But one day, when I had finally quit dieting and started living healthy, I realized that all those closetsful of clothing in assorted sizes were a Catch-22. If I kept the outfits that were too large for me, I would never be free of the safety net they provided. As the pounds started coming off, I began putting those baggy clothes into garbage bags and donating them to our local referral center (a sort of thrift shop where people can purchase needed clothing at very low prices). I think few things are harder on a person's morale than being overweight and poor, because your clothing choices are so limited, so I hoped that my donations would make someone else's life a little easier. One time Cliff had to take a whole pickup load of my clothes to the center. When he dropped the bags off, he told the people there, "I don't know how many clothes she has left at home, but if she ever gains the weight back, she's going stark naked!"

After I began setting realistic goals for myself, and I knew that I wouldn't be riding the diet roller coaster again, I also realized that I wasn't going to see size 8 or 10 again in this lifetime. With the realization that a healthy size 14 is where I belong, I then let go of all those outdated little sizes just taking up space in my storage areas.

Letting go can also mean choosing not to eat certain foods that are linked to happy memories from our pasts. We all have those "cozy" feelings about foods we loved in childhood, and while eating them again may help us relive pleasant times, it's a good time to learn to separate the happy memories from the food. The goal is to cherish the memories of those sweet times, but without succumbing to eating habits that aren't good for your health.

My strongest trigger was butter. When I was growing up in the early 1950s, my father worked in a factory, which manufactured farm tractors. My birthday is in the fall, and many times Daddy was laid off or on strike when my birthday rolled around. Money was often in short supply when it was time to celebrate, but that's a difficult thing to explain to a young child. All I wanted for my sixth birthday was a pound of real butter. I knew Mom could make something out of almost nothing, and I loved the flavor of butter so much, I wanted it to be part of the meal. My father scraped up the money for that butter somehow and my family and I thoroughly enjoyed that butter as part of my birthday supper. For twenty years after that, I ate anything that I could spread butter on. I think I would have eaten wallpaper if it was smeared with globs of butter. Then, when I was in my late twenties, we were told that butter was bad for us, so I switched to a margarine that had no cholesterol. The brand I chose tasted *almost* as good as butter, so I kept on eating two to three tubs of margarine a week. No one bothered to tell me that it was still 100 percent FAT!

When I finally started down my path to good health and began to look at the person I had become, it finally clicked. All those years, I wasn't just eating butter. I was trying to relive the fond memories of that birthday celebration. Once I made the connection, I could enjoy the memories, but I could let go of the excess amounts of unhealthy fat. Now, I buy a tub of reduced-calorie margarine, and it usually lasts me at least three months.

Sometimes we have to let go of people who stand as obstacles in our path to better health. It can be difficult distancing ourselves from those we call "friends"—until we are willing to acknowledge that they aren't treating us the ways friends do. You know who I mean. These are people who don't want you to live healthy, either because they'd rather have a "partner in crime" to make them feel better about their own unhealthy choices, or because they enjoy feeling superior about their own fit bodies and don't want you to compete with them.

This doesn't mean eliminating from your life everyone who enjoys fast food or doesn't make time to do some exercise. I'm talking about friends who may be deliberately or unconsciously sabotaging your efforts to eat and live healthy. What can you do about this? Try asking for their help, and be specific about what you want. If they truly care about you and they want what's best for you, they'll provide support as you make your way. But if they refuse your request and discourage your efforts, you can take this as a kind of wake-up call. Your time is precious and you deserve the best from those you call friends. Maybe an old friendship has run its course and no longer provides you with the sustenance that friendship should. Maybe, just maybe, it's time to let go.

An important part of letting go is making the decision to drop old habits that interfere with your goal of getting healthy. Are you still stocking the cabinets with junk food because it's always been on your shopping list, and besides, "it's for the kids"? Just think how much easier it will be on you if you aren't constantly faced with unhealthy snack foods, and how much better it will be for your family if you start buying fruit rolls and pretzels instead of high-fat cookies and candy bars.

Some habits are so ingrained, we don't even notice them—but an important part of healthy living is becoming *conscious* of what we do and how we do it. Are you still jumping in the car to run an errand that is only a few blocks' walk away? I know that driving somewhere might seem to save time, but you could "kill two birds with one stone" (or, in a computerese phrase I much prefer, try "multi-tasking" and do two things at once—exercise by walking or riding your bike, *and* pick up a prescription or mail your bills!).

What other habits can we let go of without feeling deprived? Here's a good one: Are you still "cleaning off" plates after a meal by nibbling instead of tossing the remains into the nearest garbage pail? We've all been trained to avoid waste, but turning your mouth into a handy disposal is not what your mother meant! Letting go of this unhealthy habit saves an amazing number of calories you never even knew you were eating.

Learning to recognize these habits and letting go of them is hard work, and you won't necessarily get rid of all of them the first time out. But I know that if you do the best you can one day at a time, you'll see improvement very soon.

Now we come to the most important part of letting go, but without it none of the rest will ever stay "gone." I'm talking about letting go of old beliefs that set you up for failure. Some of these beliefs are thoughts that bounce around in your own brain—worries that you won't be able to stick to your guns, fears that you've failed before at losing weight, doubts that you'll sustain your motivation to live healthy. And some of these beliefs are held by the people in your life, from your co-workers who watch what you're eating at lunch so they'll be the first to know when you "cheat" on your diet, to relatives who undercut your hard-won self-esteem by criticizing how you're doing what you're doing for yourself ("You can't eat pie for dessert and expect to keep the weight off!" "Walking won't get you thin"). How do you cope with the naysayers—those hiding in your own heads and the ones you have to deal with in person?

Ask yourself this: "Is this a belief that will let me live a better life, or will it keep me where I've been stuck for too long?" If the answer to the first is No and the second is Yes, then you know what to do—*let go of it!* Sometimes the best way to handle negativity is the same technique you use for unwelcome telemarketers who call during dinner: don't agree to be drawn into a conversation or argument, just "hang up." Say, "I appreciate your concern, but I'm doing what works for me." Say, "My doctor has okayed what I'm doing, but thanks for your advice." Stick to "just the facts," as Sergeant Joe Friday of *Dragnet* did when investigating a case. And what are the facts?

You feel better.

You look better.

Your health is improving.

Life is good.

You don't have to convince anyone but yourself. If you want to try, go ahead, but recognize that the only person you can truly influence is *you.* Let go of all that's been weighing you down, and fly!

## *A Pearl to Polish*

*I have always loved the image of the bumblebee, whose wings appear to be too small to carry his weight in flight. But seemingly in defiance of nature, the bee flies from flower to flower, nourishing itself and creating the sweet miracle of honey. When the goal before you seems out of reach, just hum quietly to yourself as you tackle the job. That soft "hmmming" will remind you that what may appear to be impossible is only just a bit beyond what you can see at that moment. It's all about letting go of the fears that hold you back.*

# Reaching Out to Others

*Nothing makes one feel so strong as a call for help.*
—GEORGE MACDONALD, AUTHOR

It feels good to belong, to fit in, to be part of something bigger than yourself. It's true whether you're in your teens or in your eighties. You're probably already part of several communities, beginning with your family. You might add to the list: your class at school, your officemates, your gym buddies, your fellow hospital volunteers, the group that decorates the church sanctuary every week. Some people are natural leaders; others seem to be natural "joiners," making time for all kinds of group activities. But others need a little push to get involved. Perhaps they're shy, or recently widowed, or feeling isolated, with small children and a husband on the road (as I often felt when Cliff worked as a long-distance trucker). Maybe they're new in town, or feeling bereft after a youngest child has left for college. Or possibly they're feeling *stuck*. (Remember how it feels to be in a rut?)

That's why I believe one of the most positive actions you can take in life is to reach out to someone else and "bring 'em along!"

I saw evidence of this in my own life when I first began creating Healthy Exchanges recipes. I would stir up healthy versions of foods I loved, and I'd bring them to my office to heat up in the microwave. As my colleagues smelled those good smells and saw that my new way of eating was helping me get healthy and feel good about myself, they asked what I was doing. Instead of keeping it to myself, I reached out and shared my recipes, shared what I'd learned about moderate exercise and making lifestyle changes. Most of all, I talked about how a change in attitude from negative to positive was transforming my life in ways I hadn't imagined!

I discovered something remarkable—that reaching out to others and sharing what worked for me helped me at the same time I was helping others. I didn't push it on anyone. I've never been known for a "hard sell," but I found that talking about what I was doing strengthened my commitment to my new lifestyle. At the same time, my healthy recipes and advice were helping my friends accomplish their own goals. Talk about a "win-win" situation!

I kept this all in mind when I created Healthy Exchanges, the company. I asked my staff to treat the people who purchased my cookbooks and the subscribers to my newsletter as "family members," not just customers. I wanted my readers to feel like an important part of what I was doing. I emphasized the idea of a Healthy Exchanges *family* because thinking of it that way helped me help others. Inviting my readers' participation and reactions, answering phone calls, and replying to e-mail brought us together on the journey to good health. I kept looking for ways to reach out and share what I'd learned, from stirring up recipes on the radio to speaking at hospitals and support groups. I got as much satisfaction from visiting with one farm wife from rural Illinois as I did appearing on QVC before a television audience of millions, because the principle was the same: Reaching out to someone else makes life better for both of us! I do a lot of my best work alone. I create recipes in the motor home while Cliff is up front driving and listening to the radio. I write my newsletter sitting at the computer in the early hours of the morning, after I've returned from a sunrise walk that filled my soul with pleasure, my heart with fresh energy, and my mind with new ideas.

Each year I go out on the road with Cliff in the RV for weeks at a time. I visit bookstores and radio stations, speak to groups and appear on TV. It's during those times that I meet my readers, my Healthy Exchange family members, and get to hear from their own lips how I've helped them make healthy changes or influenced them to get more exercise. It's exhausting and energizing at the same time! It's also immeasurably rewarding to learn that my ideas and words have touched each of them personally.

I grew up in a very small town, and I still live in one, so discovering that I've connected with so many people from all over the world still astonishes me. And all year round, between the road trips, the post office keeps delivering sacks of letters that tell me so many stories of people's lives. Plus, through the magic of e-mail, I hear from hundreds more every week!

But even with all the correspondence I've received over the years, each new encounter or hastily scribbled note feels like the first. I feel a wonderful rush of satisfaction in the knowledge that

I've had a small part in transforming a life. Reaching out does that for you, whether you're volunteering at a Red Cross blood drive or helping out at your child's school. It's empowering in a way you may not expect, and even if you don't feel you have much to offer, you *do*. When you remind a nervous young man that his single pint of blood may help save five lives, you'll make him feel like a hero (and with luck get him started on a lifelong habit!). When you listen closely to what a child says, that child will grow and flourish in the warm glow of your respect and attention. See how easy that was? It's a feeling you'll grow to like, and one you'll want to pass on to your friends and family.

I have always been grateful to God for the gift of life, but I have also discovered that through my work, I can share His most gracious gift with others. For if someone gets the tools and the strength to pursue a healthy lifestyle because of me, the gift of a better quality of life (and a longer life, too, I hope) blesses the giver as it blesses the one who receives. There is a Bible passage I have always liked that says: "Lord, make me an instrument of thy peace." *Make me an instrument . . .* I consider it my greatest accomplishment (after raising three wonderful kids!) to be an instrument of God-given good health, and I hope that I will always be blessed with that great joy.

Joy and humility filled me when a woman rushed up to me one evening, squeezed my hand, and said, "JoAnna, you literally saved my life." She was a diabetic, her blood sugar had been out of control, and her health compromised. She began cooking the Healthy Exchanges way ("food my husband would eat," she said, smiling) and in just months her condition was under control, she'd lost some weight, and she felt better than she had in years.

*It felt so good.* There's almost no way to describe the depth of emotion I feel at being able to help people help themselves. This past year has been so chaotic and at times difficult. I've been so busy, wondering if I was ever going to get it all done, and if it was all worth it anyway. So when this woman gave me the credit, I thanked her, but then I thanked God for the opportunity to make such a powerful difference in the world.

You may not feel that you have all that much to offer at this time in your life; maybe your self-esteem is a little shaky or you tend to be shy. So reaching out to others may take a real leap of faith in your value as a person. It doesn't require a college degree or years of professional experience to offer a couple of hours a week as a "baby cuddler" in a hospital, for instance. It's been proved that even the tiniest, sickest babies who are held and rocked for an extra hour a day thrive in every physical, mental, and emotional way there is. Even if you're feeling insecure about yourself, those babies won't care. They just respond to the affection that's offered.

If making the connection face-to-face isn't something you feel you can manage right now, perhaps you will decide to reach out in a more anonymous way. You can still make someone feel better about his or her life—by writing to a soldier overseas, or gathering school supplies for a distant village classroom that has very little. And via the Internet, you can participate by writing messages of hope to strangers who need a friendly word to get through a crisis. I heard the other day from Jennie, who'd been enjoying the opportunity to offer advice and comfort on a weight-loss board. Then one night, she read a note from a woman who'd been spending days and nights at the hospital with her very ill son. Feeling completely isolated and alone, she'd logged on, hoping to find some encouragement to return to a weight-loss support group—and she'd found my friend Jennie, who'd nursed her own daughter through Hodgkin's disease just a few years earlier. "All the pain I'd gone through back then now had a purpose, to enable me to reach out to this woman. With me she could open up about the fear and anger she felt, and most of all the helplessness. We exchanged e-mail addresses and we're going to keep in touch. I'm so happy to be able to be a kind of lifeline for her. It's such a blessing to be able to help someone else."

## A Pearl to Polish

*It's so easy to get caught up in our own daily efforts that we lose sight of the struggles of others. And yet many people have shared with me that they found new inspiration and energy in the act of trying to help someone else get through tough times. Others have said that simply offering advice to a person in need helped them renew their own commitment to what they were doing to help themselves. So I'm hoping you'll choose to reach out in some new way, and discover the remarkable gift that comes from giving of yourself.*

# Stay the Course

*With time and patience, the mulberry leaf becomes a silk gown.*

—CHINESE PROVERB

The late Gene Autry, that wonderful old movie cowboy, once said, "You know, if it was easy, everyone'd be doing it." I'm not exactly sure what he was referring to at the time (some difficult riding trick, perhaps?), but that doesn't really matter. I heard him and thought, "He's right. Deciding to live a healthy lifestyle, sticking to an exercise program, accentuating the positive, are worth doing. But they're not always easy. Why, if it were easy, then *everyone would be doing it*. No one would be struggling with high cholesterol or elevated blood sugar, no one would have difficulty fitting a daily workout into her schedule, and no one would ever be as much as a pound overweight!

Easy, right? Clearly not. It's not easy. It takes work. And everyone isn't doing it. But *you can*. Unlike a risky riding maneuver that takes years of practice to master, making your goal the day-to-day journey to better health is something you can tackle without a lot of training, without a hefty bankroll, without a guru to guide you—well, maybe just a grandmother with a cache of commonsense ideas about "doing it."

But "doing it" doesn't mean eating healthy for just one meal, or taking one energetic stroll through the nearest mall. "Doing it" takes commitment and time, and most of all it takes staying power. What's staying power, you may wonder? Is it like the mysterious diet aid, "willpower," that we never seem to have enough of? I think it's something else entirely, and here's why: Willpower always seems to be one of those "either/or" propositions—you either have it, or you don't. You're *on* your diet, or you're *off*. You're good—or you're not. Do you see where this is leading, down that dead-end road, *perfection?*

But none of us is perfect.

And, when faced with our imperfections, with our weaknesses, and with our lack of willpower, we often accept defeat without a struggle.

So let's put "willpower," and all that it stands for, in the back of your deepest closet or under a huge pile of dirty laundry. As an old-fashioned gangster might say, "fuggedaboudit!"

Instead, let's tackle the idea of staying power. Staying power is having the guts to stand for what you believe in when others may discourage you. Staying power is sticking by a person you love and respect even when no one else seems to be. Staying power is recognizing that, as a great philosopher once put it, "success is one percent inspiration, ninety-nine percent perspiration." Staying power proves the old adage that the most important ingredient for success is *just showing up.*

Okay. So you're here and you're feeling really motivated today. Good for you. You're pumped up, you're ready to roll. But what about those mornings when the sky is gray, you're not in the mood to get up and walk, or it feels like just too much trouble to prepare a healthy meal when the telephone number for pizza delivery is looking mighty attractive there on the refrigerator?

Aha. Time to call on that old *staying power.* Make a little deal with yourself. Maybe say, "Get up and turn on all the lights in the house, and you can have pancakes for breakfast." (You can, after all. It's the piles of butter and sugary syrup that aren't great for you.) Or, "Pull on your sweats, tie those shoelaces, and walk for just five minutes. If by then you're still feeling crummy, you can come back." (I've tried this. It's amazing how just five minutes is enough to get you feeling more "up" about exercise!) Or you might try negotiating: "Instead of ordering pizza now when I'm home alone and might feel tempted to devour the whole pie, why not invite some friends over this weekend for a pizza party?"

Staying power is about not giving up on yourself. It's about searching for a solution that can meet your emotional needs and still keep you on the road to feeling good about yourself. It's about making a commitment to do the best you can today, and to show up again tomorrow, determined to doing your best once more.

Some days, your best is just spectacular. You put in extra minutes at the gym, you eat crunchy, healthy salads for lunch *and* dinner, you look at yourself in the mirror and say, "I look gooooood!"

Some days, your best is just showing up. Just getting out of bed, making a little time for a walk, choosing the best options you can find on a restaurant menu, and being kind to yourself and others.

And some days, you don't consider that what you've done is anywhere near "your best." On those days, maybe you skipped your workout. On those days, maybe you gobbled down a couple of cookies during your break at work. On those days, maybe you found fault with your appearance every time you passed a store window. . . . or perhaps your mother-in-law or husband did.

On those days, all you want to do is run away, to hide—with a box of chocolates if at all possible. Feel the impulse, recognize why you feel that way, and then whisper to yourself, "Stay." Say it again, a little louder this time. Now, one last time in a firm voice: "Stay." Take a couple of deep breaths, and hold that thought for a minute.

*Stay.* Stand and fight for what you truly want. You want to be healthy, to feel good about yourself. You want to go on, not quit. You would gladly defend your best friend or your sister if someone criticized her for her failings. Now it's time to do the same for yourself!

A longtime friend of mine shared with me that she loved the support of a weight-loss group and did extremely well as long as she went to the weekly meetings. "I like offering helpful ideas to the other women in the class," Suzanne said. "Every time I raise my hand, it's like I get a shot of adrenaline and a positive push that keeps me on the right track."

But then she added, "That's great, until I have a bad week

and think I won't lose any weight—or will even gain. So I skip that class, vowing I'll do better next week and return, but I don't, and the bad weeks start adding up. Soon, I've gained back everything I lost and then some. Sometimes it takes years before I try again." Suzanne knows what works for her, but when she is less than perfect, she tends to silence the little voice in her ear that whispers, "Stay. Stay no matter what kind of week you've had. Stay and keep fighting for what you want. Stay and enjoy the rush of positive energy you get by helping others. Stay, and give yourself a fresh start, a new beginning. Oh, just stay!"

When I asked her if I could include her story in this chapter, she agreed, because she's recently made a new commitment to herself. She's back at her group, she's feeling more motivated than she has in years, and she's hung signs with the word *Stay* all over her apartment to reinforce the idea that it's important to stick with what works, even during times of struggle and disappointment.

So—even when you're feeling discouraged, or when the needle on the scale won't move, or you feel you can't eat another piece of fruit this week, *stay*. Stay with me on the Health Wagon, ride alongside friends heading in the same direction. Oh, we may hit a bump or two, or even break an axle. But I promise you, we're sharing the same journey, and you're not alone.

### A Pearl to Polish

*When I asked Michelle, who'd chosen a marathon as her goal, how anyone could run 26.2 miles, she replied it was possible only because she never focused on the entire thing. She knew she could run for a half hour, so that would cover about three miles. Then she thought about the next chunk of it. Before she knew it, an hour had passed, and she'd covered six miles. "I just kept carving off little chunks of the distance, enjoying the scenery, visiting with other runners near me, and listening to my radio," she said. "I walked a little in the later stages, but when I realized I had three miles to go, I thought, 'I can run three miles any day.' That thought kept me going until the finish line was in sight."*

By focusing on what she could do, on manageable amounts of a task that seemed impossible when considered in its entirety, Michelle reached a goal that she'd once believed was out of her reach. The secret was that she stayed, kept putting one foot in front of the other, until she got where she'd dreamed of going.

The great scientist Louis Pasteur wrote, "Let me tell you of the secret that has led me to my goal. My strength lies solely in my tenacity."

# Put Your Body in Motion, Your Mind Will Follow

*Even if you're on the right track, you'll still get run over if you just sit there.*

—WILL ROGERS

If you studied Latin in school (I didn't, but I have friends who did), you might already know that the word *inspiration* comes from a word that means "breathe." So it makes perfect sense to me that anyone on the path to better health will find inspiration through activities that require a little (or a lot of) deep breathing!

One of the reasons I was oh-so-ready to change my prayer from losing weight to living healthy was a genuine difficulty breathing. It scared me that I woke up at night because of a condition called sleep apnea, in which you actually stop breathing for an instant or two. It also scared me that walking up a flight of stairs left me gasping for breath. If I'd still been a mother of young children, I don't think I would have been able to run after them, lift and carry them, perhaps even keep them safe.

When I began living a healthy lifestyle, most people could see the outward changes in my body as I started losing weight. But what they couldn't see and probably didn't even think about was my commitment to moderate exercise, which for me consisted mostly of walking briskly, riding my bike, or splashing around aerobically in the pool at the Hart Center, our local health club.

Well, in a world where grandmothers in their seventies are running marathons, my fitness efforts probably didn't warrant a second glance from anyone outside my immediate family. But my exercise efforts, coupled with my weight loss, began a transformation in me that continues to this very day.

Yes, my symptoms of sleep apnea and breathlessness disappeared over time, and for that I was extremely grateful. But what I found more "inspiring" was how I began to feel every single day. I could breathe better, more deeply, expanding my lungs and feeling my shoulders relax as I drew in much more air than I ever had before. Many people who are overweight tend to breathe shallowly, inhaling the bare minimum of air they need to feel good. Not getting enough air has a real impact on how you feel, and finally exhaling all the carbon dioxide my body couldn't use and replacing it with lots of fresh oxygen energized my body from head to toe!

The sensation was pretty amazing, and as I continued in my journey to better health, I paid attention to how my moderate exercise and my deeper breathing influenced the way I tackled my day, the ease with which I fell asleep at night, the vim and vigor I felt when I got out of bed each morning, and the stamina I discovered I had to carry me through a whirlwind of daily activities.

Exercise, I learned through my own experience, wasn't just good for the heart. The act of moving my limbs while walking or bike riding, even though I wasn't particularly fast, challenged my lungs to exchange old air for new and opened up the pores of my skin through healthy perspiration, so I could clear my system of impurities when I showered afterward. While I've always been known for my rosy complexion, my skin truly glowed when I was getting some physical exercise on a regular basis. No woman needs more encouragement than that to keep doing what's working, and so, too, was I "inspired" to put my body in motion just about every day.

I found another fascinating aspect of the power of exercise when I paid attention to how what I was doing made me look and feel. When my day was particularly stressful and I was tempted to skip my ride or walk because it was harder than usual to find the time, I realized that by making myself "go through the motions" at the start, I could be aware of a remarkable amount of the stress I was under. And by promising myself just to do a little something (and that I could stop if it got too cold or began pouring or whatever), I noticed that just getting myself "out the door" made a world of difference. If I could just make myself lace on my sneakers or buckle on my Teva sandals, I could get myself out the door. And if I could just get myself out the door, I could persuade myself to keep going for a few minutes, at least.

Once those few minutes had passed, I nearly always kept going because I started to feel so much better than when I had begun. The running magazines call this the "endorphin effect," where after a certain number of minutes of exercising, the body has a tendency to release "feel-good" hormones that sustain your efforts. Your body wants you to keep moving it and keep it healthy, and so it provides a little hormonal encouragement to persuade you to go, go, go! Even if the mind isn't convinced, the body provides a kind of "override" that says, "Yes, you can—Yes, you should—Yes!"

Even when you're engaged in physical activity that has nothing to do with "exercise" per se, your body can be very encouraging in ways you don't even notice. Remember the last time you went dancing with your husband or partner, and you felt so good you just never wanted to leave the floor? You danced the slow ones and the fast ones, and when you woke up the next morning you may even have been a little stiff because of the exertion. But oh, my, while you were dancing, you felt just like Eliza Doolittle in the musical *My Fair Lady*. You really could have danced all night!

It's the same with exertion that takes place in beautiful environments that inspire the heart and soul even as the body feels endlessly motivated to keep moving. I've heard people marvel at how on a given day they were able to hike up a mountain with family members, even if they usually found themselves out of breath after a couple of flights of stairs. One woman wrote to me about exceeding all her expectations for success when she agreed to be part of a team raising money for breast cancer. For her, that meant walking more than a hundred miles over several days. "I was inspired," she told me, and I believe it. But I also credit that sneaky body of hers, which so loved breathing deeply for hours on end that it wanted more!

For all these reasons, I'm a real stickler for making moderate exercise part of any healthy living program, whether you're hoping to lose weight, lower your cholesterol, strengthen a recovering heart, or get your blood sugar under control. There are astonishing health benefits to moving even just a little bit, and not all of them are physical. Sometimes the most powerful benefit of putting your body in motion is the psychological lift you get by simply "going through the motions." To lift your foot to take a step, you need air, and when you draw a deep breath to provide your body with that oxygen, you lift yourself at the same time.

You lift your heart with a kind of secret pleasure that you're doing something good for yourself. You lift your soul because making a physical effort can provide a surprising spiritual link to the Lord and to the nature He created. You lift your mind in new hope that doing this one little thing for yourself can make a difference between feeling depressed about your health and feeling optimistic about how you can improve it.

You even get a sensual lift when you walk, or jog, or bike, or dance, or row, or jump rope, or swim. Your eyes see the beauty of flowers as you walk down a country road. Your nose inhales the sweet aroma of freshly mowed grass as you ride your bike through your quiet neighborhood in the morning. Your ears are filled with the song of birds and the clicks of crickets as you jog through town after sunset. Your lips smile at your partner as you dance up a storm. And your entire body feels a rush of pleasure as you glide through the deep blue water of the pool.

But even on those days when you're not in the mood, or when it's raining too hard to walk outside, or the snow is too deep to ride your bike, if you find some way to put your body in motion, your mind and spirit are sure to follow. As the body goes through the rhythmic motions, the brain is free to wander—and anything is possible. You may find yourself composing a poem in your head, or you may get a fantastic idea for your son's Halloween costume.

Your stressed-out mind may relax enough to engineer the perfect solution to a problem that's been bothering you all day.

And if your baby just won't stop crying, it's possible that she needs a walk or a ride, too, but she doesn't yet know how to ask for it. As the stroller wheels start turning, her frowns turn to smiles and the transformation is complete. A little "inspiration" is good for everyone—even the dog!

### A Pearl to Polish

*Most of us get into fitness ruts in our lives. We use the same machines at the gym, we walk the same routes from our houses to the store, and we begin to believe that our workout is the only one that "works." If you're feeling uninspired (there's that word again!), change your path and try something new. If you always walk for exercise, add a spurt of race-walking between lightposts every couple of blocks. Change your bike route so it includes a hill (or if you can't find one, pretend every few minutes or so that you're riding uphill and have to pump harder). If you always swim the crawl or freestyle, try alternating those laps with breaststroke for a change. Inspiration is all about fresh breath, and sometimes the only way to find it is to change what you're doing.*

# Seeds of Faith

---

*Ask, and it shall be given you; seek, and ye shall find; knock,*
*and it shall be opened unto you.*

—JESUS

*F*aith is at the heart of who I am, and it has shaped my life in a hundred big and small ways. Believing in what you cannot see, committing to a process whose end is uncertain, requires a kind of trust that must be learned but cannot really be taught. I learned something of what it meant to be a person of faith at home from the time I was a small child. It wasn't just about going to church or believing in what the minister taught me, though surely we are the sum total of all our experiences, including what we take from the services we attend.

I think my grandmother Carrington, my mother's mother, made the strongest impression on me. She was a perfect example of teaching by doing what was right, not teaching by preaching about it. If you needed help, Annie Carrington would be there for you, no questions asked. My grandmother wasn't a public person, not someone looking for special attention. Her life was a simple one—she cooked for her boarders at the boarding house, nourishing their soul and bodies, caring for her "extended family" as warmly as she did her relatives. As I grew older, I began to understand the depth of her commitment to these people, how she drew them to her table and kept them in her heart.

I will never forget one particular way my grandmother taught me about faith, and about reaching out to others. There were three young boys in her town, teenagers whose parents had abandoned them. She took them in and let them help around the farm, made them part of the family. As they grew older, they just stayed and stayed, and my grandparents in effect became their parents. Plenty of people in the community clucked and said, "How awful," but no one else came forward to help.

Those boys were always there, part of our lives, and even though they came and went as they grew older, they always came back. One even stayed with my grandmother until the day she died, and it was he who finally closed the boarding house. Those boys responded to her unselfish and generous love in kind, offering affection and even financial support over the years. For me, it was a wonderful example of living your faith. The "seed" of her example grew in all her children and grandchildren, and I see it today in my own kids as well. My parents and my aunt and uncle were much the same way, and even as a young girl I became aware of the difference between observing need from a distance and doing something about it. I come from a family of big-hearted people, and I'm proud of how they practiced their faith in all they did.

So I consider myself just the latest in a long family tradition of planting seeds of faith. I always wanted to do justice to this legacy in a way I know would please my grandmother. The mail I receive daily and the stories I hear when I'm on the road tell me that I'm carrying on what Grandma taught me—planting seeds of faith and hope in gardens I may never get to see.

Sometimes, though, I'm lucky enough to share in a bit of the bounty of that spiritual harvest. Recently, I met a woman who was particularly grateful for the life changes she'd been en-couraged to make after reading my HELP book. She told me that I had *neshama,* a Hebrew word for soul that I later discovered has a wonderful and even deeper meaning. The teachings of Judaism say that it's not enough just to study and learn and live a good life, but that it pleases the Lord best when you reach out and teach others what you have learned, planting seeds of faith and belief in the possibility of change.

This woman's words meant a great deal to me, told me that I was fulfilling my "ministry" as I had set out to do so long ago. It had been immensely satisfying to set difficult goals like losing a lot of weight and regaining my health, but I'd known almost from the start that I wouldn't be satisfied with just focusing on my own problems. I discovered that the power I'd found inside myself to create such changes in my life only grew stronger when I offered what I'd found to others. Transforming my own "soul's journey" into a shared one gave me new insights into my own heart, and it allowed me to make connections with others who were looking for guidance on their own path.

Interestingly, this gift of faith, of being able to help others find a new way to live, seems to be transferable. I've heard from many people over the years, men and women who've done more than simply succeed in reaching their own goals of better health and losing weight. In each case, they became determined to "share the wealth" of information and motivation they'd found. And so they were offering healthy cooking classes at their churches, or speaking to community groups about getting started on a walking program. Some decided to go back to school to be teachers or fitness trainers; others simply passed along healthy recipes at the office to colleagues who'd noticed the changes they'd made and found the courage to ask for help.

It takes a certain kind of courage to own up to your own success, to be willing to put yourself on the line with others and suggest ways of changing their lives for the better. It requires faith in yourself and what you've accomplished—perhaps the ultimate form of the positive attitude I encourage in everything I write.

It also takes a firm faith to stick to your guns when everyone around you is touting some hot new diet or heavily promoted body-shaping machine. Following the crowd has always been easier, but the result of doing what everyone else tells you to do is often not the result you want. So nurturing the seeds of your faith in what you're doing is important, especially when your true goal is sustaining change over the months and years ahead.

Faith by definition is hard to pin down. In part, it means believing in what you can't see, and that can be hard when you're as practical and down-to-earth as I try to be. But it's also about believing in what can't be measured with spoons, cups, or scales—like doing your best to raise your children with good judgment and character, then having the confidence to send those kids off to college without fearing they will forget the lessons you've taught. You begin planting seeds of faith from the moment a child arrives, and you can't be certain of the results for many years. But by focusing on what you believe is good and true, you prepare your children to experience the world—and you hope that what you've taught them will sustain them through challenging and difficult times.

It's easier to see how the seeds of faith in others flourish, and less obvious to us how the seeds of our own faith are growing. We commit to an education, not knowing just how all those years of classes will develop our minds and transform our lives. We choose a career for any one of a hundred reasons, uncertain that it's the right choice but determined to make it work. We may decide to share our lives with romantic partners, knowing only a little about the people they are and even less about who they will someday become. We take so very much on faith, hoping to nurture the seeds of our trust in the future into something beautiful and strong.

### A Pearl to Polish

*Why have faith in what we cannot see, cannot measure, cannot touch or lock away in a safe place? Why believe in the promises made by our parents, our teachers, our clergy, when the world seems such an uncertain place?*

*Why, indeed? So much of what is most meaningful in our lives is invisible, and yet we would not choose to live without it. Love . . . happiness . . . courage . . . kindness . . . hope . . . these are the touchstones of a good life, and we take them on faith. So, too, must we take on faith our belief that we have the strength and power to shape our own future. With each change we make, each choice and each commitment, we change what is inevitable into what is possible. We grow, just as seeds in a garden do, with a lot of water, a lot of love, and a lot of faith.*

# Making Mistakes, Then Making Some More

*You are making progress if each mistake you make is a new one.*

—ANONYMOUS

$O$ne of my favorite things about having a Healthy Exchanges website is the opportunity it's provided for my HE family members to share their thoughts and encourage each other as they travel the road to better health. When I have a free moment, I peek into the various folders to see what people are sharing, and to hear what their concerns are. Often I'll read something that will spark an idea or help me choose a theme for a future newsletter column. It may be just a few words that hit home for me, and I hope the same is true for other visitors.

Here's an inspiring message from one of my wonderful correspondents: Pat welcomed a recent arrival to the site and encouraged her to keep trying. Then she wrote: "This is not a 'diet'—it's about learning to make healthy choices. I guess I don't feel so bad when I make a 'wrong' choice; I learn to make better ones in the future. . . . Keep up the good choices and leave the bad ones in the dust. They say it takes two weeks to establish a new 'habit'—hang in there!"

Do you remember how it felt to start a new diet? You emptied the cabinets of all temptations, bought lots of veggies, vowed to drink water, and promised yourself to follow the menu perfectly. Secretly you knew there was really no other choice—either you were perfect and "on," or you were cheating and "off." And once you cheated even a tiny bit or ate the wrong thing by mistake, your inner binger was off and running! After all, just as you can't be a little bit pregnant, you can't be less than perfectly perfect—or you're not perfect at all!

Well, I'm not perfect and, I'd be willing to bet, neither are you. We're all human and we all make mistakes. We slip, we slide, we nibble without thinking, we celebrate joyful occasions, and we cope with tragic events. If I was Saint JoAnna, then I wouldn't have to worry about that spoonful of shortcake or that forkful of bread pudding. I'd be perfect.

But I'm not a saint, and I won't ever be. Instead, I'm a woman who's trying her best every day to live healthy and make good choices when it comes to food, exercise, self-esteem, and relationships. Does that sound familiar? I hope so. Because when I write my books and newsletters, the readers I imagine are people a lot like me: women and men with a lot on their plates when it comes to work and family, but who are committed to doing the best they can, *the best they can,* each and every day of their lives. Some days, they do better than others. Some days, so do I.

Being human and living a full life means making decisions—and making decisions, hundreds of them every day, means
making mistakes. It's normal, it's natural, and for most of us, it's
how we learn and grow. Remember the first time someone told
you about the multiplication tables? You knew the basics of how
to add and subtract, and as long as the numbers were small, you
could double-check on your fingers and toes. But oh my goodness, *multiplication?* You had to memorize, take things on faith,
believe that if two times four is eight, that six times four is
twenty-four! Maybe the first few times, while you were still
learning, and the teacher asked you, "How much is six times
four?" you hesitated, calculated the best you could, but still
weren't sure what the answer was. It came with time, and practice, and study.

Well, making the changes to a healthier lifestyle is another
learning experience—maybe one of the most important ones of
your life. But you shouldn't expect to know it all the first day or
the first week, or even the first month. Learning to read took lots
of time, but it was worth it. Well, this will be too.

Many of the letters I get from new readers express concern
that they won't get it "right," that because they're not absolutely
certain how to use the exchanges or to use their optional calories
something awful will happen. I spend a lot of time reassuring
them that they can learn to follow the program. But more than
that, I want them to see that change occurs one day at a time, and
often it's best not to try to absorb *everything* at once. Instead, you
want to focus on the habits that got you where you are, and how
you're going to make positive changes, to exchange old habits for

new healthy ones when it comes to food, exercise, and mental attitude.

Most people focus first on learning a new way of eating, but I recommend that they first try to cope with the anxiety and stress that may come with making a fresh start. I remind them that their common sense will carry them through these confusing early stages, but I always add that of course they will make mistakes.

The quotation I chose to start this chapter with is a heartfelt one: Try hard not to repeat your mistakes, but recognize that most learning occurs through trial and error. Yes, of course, you can study hard and you may have the basics of the program down quite fast. But then you may have a day when you're stressed-out, you're stuck eating somewhere that makes choosing difficult, you're faced with unexpected events that keep you from your regular exercise schedule, and *bam*—old fears will surface and you'll think that whatever was working for you is now lost.

It's *not*. Tell yourself, that meal is over. That frustrating day is over. That party with all the temptations is over. The person who kept pressuring you to eat, eat, eat is gone. Now, you've got a new day and new chances to make good choices. Remember, a mistake you don't learn from is wasted time (and calories!).

On the other hand, living a safe dieter's life is another kind of mistake. Skipping parties so you can eat dry tuna and lettuce leaves at home is a mistake. Turning down a dinner invitation because you might have to choose from an unfamiliar menu is a mistake. Being afraid to go on a cruise or other vacation because you might overeat is a mistake as well. Don't let your fear of making a mistake limit the variety of your life experiences—these are some of the pleasures that make life worth living. A party isn't only about food; it's also about meeting new people, dancing, and celebrating. An invitation to dinner is a manageable risk, and an opportunity to broaden your world. As for a cruise—most of the beautiful ships that travel the world's oceans provide just as many chances to exercise and stay active as they do to eat, so why would you deny yourself the excitement of Alaska or the sultry breezes of the Caribbean?

## A Pearl to Polish

*Making mistakes is part of everyday life, and accepting that it's nearly impossible to be perfect is an important step on the road to loving self-acceptance. One of the most serious mistakes people make is being unwilling to try what they fear they won't excel at. Think of it this way: A scientist who fears being wrong will never succeed in finding the cure for anything, and an explorer who fears making a mistake will never discover new lands. There's a wonderful quote I heard once that says, "In order to discover new oceans, you have to be willing to lose sight of the shore."*

*Keep that thought in mind as you take more of life's risks, whether you're meeting new people, attempting an unfamiliar sport, or choosing to follow a new healthy-living plan. Even while you are feeling adrift, with no visible landmarks to help you navigate, you're on your way to discovering new worlds of experience and knowledge.*

# Winning Your Angel Wings

---

*I shall not pass this way again; let me now relieve some pain, remove some barrier from the road, or lighten someone's heavy load.*

—EVA ROSE YORK, AUTHOR AND COMPOSER

$\mathcal{M}$ost dieters have experienced the sensation of lightness that comes with weight loss. When the vanished pounds mount up and the scale keeps moving down, you're literally carrying less weight around, so it's natural that you might find a new quickness to your step, less achiness in your shoulders, even a remarkable absence of morning pain in your feet. (That was one of my worst problems when I was at my highest weight—I'd crawl out of bed and actually have to balance on the sides of my feet for the first few minutes, because it hurt so much to walk on my soles!)

Even when the pounds lost amount to only one or two, there's a psychological feeling of lightness, especially when you pick up a pound of butter in the supermarket and realize you're not "wearing" it anymore. Or you lift a two-pound can of tomatoes and discover with stunned surprise how much two pounds actually is. Even if you've got a long way to get near your goal weight, by acknowledging the physical reality of *any* loss, you're likely to enjoy at least a little bit of "loft"!

But there's so much more to the kind of lightening up I have in mind. Even before the pounds start coming off, I want to encourage you to "lighten up" on yourself. Many overweight people who've tried time after time to lose weight and keep it off tend to be very hard on themselves. That kind of critical self-view weighs heavily on the soul, and when the soul is weighed down, it's so much harder to make the kind of positive changes in your life that will lead to long-term weight loss and improved health.

What do I mean when I ask you to lighten up?

First, I hope you will become aware of how you treat yourself, how you view your body, and what kind of self-talk you use. When someone asks you how you're feeling or doing, do you say (without thinking, in an old, not very positive, habit): "I'm feeling fat today. I'm having a bad hair day. Nothing I'm doing seems to be working"? Those kinds of comments bring back some pretty unfortunate memories for me, so I figure you're not unfamiliar with them, either. Psychologists have told me that the brain "hears" what you say when you repeat such negative self-descriptions aloud, and it incorporates them in your psyche. That's why so many therapists and self-help programs talk about the power of positive affirmations to transform your mind and body. Imagine how you might feel if instead of the negative answers above, you replied, "When the sun is shining so brightly, I feel like anything is possible. My hair had a mind of its own this morning, and I decided to go with a new look. Seeing you always makes me feel good—how are you?"

Feel any lighter? It's amazing but true!

When you surround yourself with a cloak of positive attitude, a sense that you can control your destiny (which has only a little to do with the size of your thighs), you've already begun to lighten up on yourself—and your body will respond by lightening up on you!

Part of the inspiration for this chapter came from a lovely note card someone sent me that was created by illustrator Mary Engelbreit. The inspiring cover line on the card (written by S. Levine) says, "Angels can fly because they take themselves so lightly!" That image just stuck in my imagination, and I began thinking about how it might really feel to fly, to leave the earth behind and move through space with your heart lifted and your shoulders relaxed, your eyes bright with excitement and your soul free as a bird to dream of going anywhere.

Have you ever felt that free? It's a fantasy, of course, but there are definitely steps we can all take to release what holds us down and back from living as fully and freely as possible. Positive self-talk is probably the first and best way to lighten up on yourself, in part because it's so easy to get started, and you've got so many opportunities in any given day. Your boss drops a pile of unexpected work on your desk, and your first impulse is to feel angry, overburdened, unappreciated. "What does she expect of me?" you may start muttering bitterly, and all of a sudden your lower back begins to ache, your neck stiffens up, and you feel every one of your extra forty pounds pressing on your spine. The emotional negativity you've just experienced provokes an almost immediate physical reaction, and your energy level sinks to its lowest ebb. But suppose you'd just decided that today you'd begin lightening up on yourself—and instead you looked at the new stack of papers and said aloud, "She can't get along without me. I'm instrumental to her success, and it's good to know that she depends so much on me. Before I tackle this mess, I'm going to take an early lunch, go for a walk outside, and hmm, maybe buy some grapes to snack on while I'm slaving away this afternoon." By choosing to focus on what is positive in the situation, and by deciding that you have some control over how you orchestrate your day, you feel an emotional lift, a sense of pride comes over you, and you stand up and march down the hall with a bit of extra oomph in your stride.

Turning negative reactions around is only one way to begin lightening up on yourself. Another might be deciding to give up feeling guilty all the time. I identified so with Nancy when she e-mailed me, saying, "Guilt is driving me crazy. I feel guilty when I eat something I like, even if it's a healthy piece of cheesecake, because for years my mother criticized every bite of food that went into my mouth. Now she's gone, but I still hear her saying, 'Should you be eating that?' when I bring the fork to my lips! And that's not all. I feel guilty when I leave the dishes in the sink while I go for a walk after dinner, and I feel guilty when I turn down a colleague's invitation to lunch because I'd rather go to the gym instead. I even get the "guilts" when I ask my husband to fold his own socks while he's watching TV so I can get to a yoga class. All this guilt is exhausting, but I don't seem to be able to talk myself out of it!"

Nancy, you're not alone. Guilt in some form weighs down most of the women I've spoken with over the years. We've learned to put ourselves and our needs last, in many cases because our mothers were so self-sacrificing and we thought it was the only acceptable way to be. Now, of course, we're paying the price in extra pounds, high blood pressure, stress-related illnesses, and exhaustion. Unfortunately, the only way to change things is for us to declare our independence from the guilt that drains us of the energy we need to live our lives well. We succumb to guilt because we care what other people think more than we care about our own best instincts; we struggle to live up to everyone's expectations of us before we commit to putting our own hopes and dreams first. But no one else can banish the guilt from our hearts and minds—we've got to do it ourselves.

The simple truth is, there isn't enough time to do everything we *want* to do and everything we think we *should* do. Something's got to give, and I suggest we start with the "shoulds." This doesn't mean refusing to drive your share of the car pool, but it could mean getting other parents to pitch in more and take some of the burden off you. It could mean reorganizing your household so your kids take on more chores than they're used to doing. And it could mean learning to accept that the house might not be as spotless, or that your reputation as someone who will always pitch in or stay late might have to change. But giving up some of those extra responsibilities may produce qualms of guilt. Are you letting people down who used to count on you? Maybe, but is that more important than possibly letting yourself down? If you can learn to live with being a little less perfect, a little less available, and a lot less of a pushover, you will likely find more time for the things that matter most to you—and at the same time feel much better about yourself!

How about some other ways to lighten up on yourself? You've already tackled negative self-talk; you're going to try to give up guilt; you're thinking about surrendering some of the responsibilities you've taken on that have grown to be too much. Hmm—what else could you do?

How about putting aside old expectations of how you expect to look and feel? Are you still hoping to squeeze back into a size-6 dress you wore on your honeymoon, even though you're now a grandmother and married nearly half a century? Do you have a magic number in mind—the perfect weight that has always been your impossible dream—and nothing less will do? Do you carry around a twenty-year-old photograph of yourself and keep comparing the woman in the mirror to the lady in the picture with not a wrinkle or crow's foot in sight?

Sometimes what weighs us down in the present is a longing to reclaim our past selves. Instead of setting more realistic goals, we fantasize about wiping years away by crash-dieting or working out to exhaustion or by spending lots of hard-earned money on skin-care products that promise eternal youth. But while motivating yourself with an image that recalls a fitter, healthier you isn't wrong, it can be self-defeating to expect to achieve such results—and in most cases, fail. I heard from a lady in the Northeast who stopped in the middle of cleaning out her closets to bring me up to date on her progress. Annie wrote, "I'm so happy with how I look and feel, but I've finally had to accept that I won't be wearing the dresses I saved from ten years ago. Yes, I can fit into them, and that's great, but they look so dated now. I kept them all this time because they represented the possibility of getting back down to a size 12, but now that I'm there, I see that they're part of the past and it's time to let them go." With that understanding, Annie lightened up on herself by setting aside expectations from the past. She's ready to live in the real world now, and to see herself in clothes that suit the woman she is today, not the woman she was a decade in the past.

Are you carrying around old expectations of how you hope to look? Are your closets stuffed with smaller-size garments you've been saving for a better day? Are you coloring your hair the same dark shade it was when you were twenty-five? Maybe it's time to lighten up on yourself by seeing yourself as you are now, and making that person look as beautiful and healthy as you can. What looked good on you when you were younger may not suit you anymore, and even if it means donating some barely worn dresses and suits to the charity thrift shop, it can be so much better to live for today in every way.

### A Pearl to Polish

*What weighs more, a pound of iron or a pound of feathers? For a moment, you think, well, iron is so heavy, it's just got to weigh more than feathers, right? Feathers are light and soft, birds fly with them, how heavy could they be? Ah, but we all know this trick question! A pound is a pound, after all, and a pound of feathers weighs the same as a pound of iron. Two people may weigh the same number on the scale, but one may plod through life as if she were wearing a pair of iron clogs, while the other seems to have wings on her feet. The difference between them? A decision to lighten up. Just for today, imagine you've been touched by an angel, and your sneakers have wings instead of weights. As you experience a bouncier step and a lighter heart, that angel's touch will help you learn to fly free!*

# Getting Focused and Staying Focused

*Only when your consciousness is totally focused on the moment you are in can you receive whatever gift, lesson, or delight that moment has to offer.*

—BARBARA DE ANGELIS, AUTHOR

*O*n an average day, my phone rings about every thirty seconds. Someone knocks on the door of my office about every five minutes, and between those interruptions I receive frequent beeps on the intercom asking me to answer "just one quick question."

It's a wonder I get anything done.

This list doesn't even include other kinds of necessary or unnecessary pauses: The bell rings on the oven timer; the doorbell rings with a delivery; Cliff wants to ask about plans for an upcoming book tour; a workman needs an answer on something related to the house; a radio station wants five minutes with me for a morning show. . . .

You get the picture. Sometimes, all it takes is a loud noise to break your concentration. Other times, it may be an urgent need to visit the rest room. As the wonderful Gilda Radner used to have her Roseanne Roseannadanna character say on *Saturday Night Live,* "It's always something!"

*Yes, it is.*

Now, I could scream and shout and plead that I need quiet to write my next newsletter or to create the perfect recipe for an upcoming occasion or to make notes for a speech I'm giving at a seminar or event. (And I won't deny that I haven't ever done so!) But at some point I have to recognize that I don't inhabit a perfectly noise-free, controlled environment, and that I live not in isolated peacefulness (even in my small Iowa town) but in the thick of things. The world won't stop because I have work to do, so I must find a way to function in the midst of what often feels like chaos.

For most people, figuring out how to handle this problem is an ongoing concern. And for most people, there is no one easy answer or system or solution that provides complete satisfaction. But it's important to acknowledge that there is a problem that needs solving, and to do something to try to make it better. If what you try doesn't work, you may at least acquire some insight into another way to tackle the challenge. At least you have the satisfaction that you're doing *something* instead of throwing in the towel and signing yourself into the local mental health center!

I think the first step in tackling a problem is narrowing it down, and so I always try to zero in on what is most important or time-sensitive. When I used to answer all my own phone calls, I found it hard to keep promising I'd call people back, so I'd usually just keep taking every call. Nowadays, though, when my Healthy Exchanges staff answers the phone, I've got a bit of a cushion in place. If I'm working on a deadline, they already know that I want to be interrupted only if: (1) it's any of my children or Cliff; (2) it's one of my publishing colleagues, whose busy schedules echo my own; or (3) it's truly urgent or an emergency that can't wait. Otherwise, they take a message, promising to put it in my hands as soon as I'm free. My caller doesn't feel slighted but recognizes that I want to give her or him my full attention. Instead of getting half a minute with a scatterbrain who's got one eye on the computer screen and the other on a pile of correspondence on her desk, they'll get a focused and thoughtful me—and we'll accomplish much more.

I don't expect you to hire a receptionist to screen your calls when you're doing something important, unless, of course, your own home business has evolved to require one! But a phone machine can work wonders in limiting interruptions and providing a real opportunity for you to focus on what is important to you. This is even true when all you have planned is a relaxing bath to de-stress after a busy day. By setting even modest limits on your availability, you will discover a sense of control you may feel your life has lacked for ages.

What if you're drowning in papers and can't find what you need when you need it? Erika, a writer friend of mine, always talks about the flood of mail, clippings, and "to-do" lists that pile up in her home and office. She told me, "If I don't see it, I don't do it. So even though I keep a calendar of appointments in my Filofax, I also have a magnetized file folder attached to the back of my front door. That's where I keep what I want to remember when leaving the house: schedules for volunteer work, tickets for events, even coupons that must be used this week. Every time I open the door to bring in the paper or head out on an errand, my eyes roam over what's posted. I feel as if I have a personal assistant handing me exactly what I need to get done."

Hmm, getting things done. Take a moment to think about your style of accomplishing what you want and need to do. Are you in a constant state of feeling overwhelmed because you can't find the time or the project at hand seems much too big? Many books on getting organized suggest nibbling away at big jobs and breaking them down into manageable segments. I've done this myself, and I know it works. But I'm also a fan of declaring a family day of decluttering, when everyone pitches in to tackle a major task together. If the garage is so full that the cars don't fit in there anymore, it's not your problem; it's a family problem, and requires a group effort. Why? Because the problem isn't a messy, overcrowded space—well, not just that. It's a systems issue, a chance to answer two important questions: How did it get that way? How can we discourage it from happening again once we dig out?

The other reason it involves everyone is that everyone's "stuff" is part of the problem. There was a popular slogan back in the sixties: "If you're not part of the solution, you're part of the problem." By getting everyone to participate in determining the solution, you make a tremendous amount of headway in solving the problem once and for all!

But what if you're having difficulty getting and staying focused because of the job itself? You have to write a paper but you just can't get started? You need to clean out your late mother's attic but something comes up every time you plan to do it? You know you need to have your house painted but the idea of packing up your entire collection of Carnival glass, along with everything else in the house, seems like more than you can stand?

Believe me, I know the feeling of being paralyzed by a big task. We all do.

Being stuck takes your focus away from what you need to get done. Your stress level increases with each passing day. You have trouble falling asleep, you feel edgy and even angry, and you react negatively to the slightest disagreement with your spouse or your kids. You know you have to do something. But even contemplating the job shoves your blood pressure upward. Yet the longer you let the struggle continue, the harder it becomes to act. Finally, it comes down to a moment of truth: Is it more painful to stay where you are, in the state you're in, or to tackle what you've been resisting for so long?

Sometimes it helps me to make lists on both sides of the issue: not just what's the worst that will happen if I do it, or if I don't, but also, and much more important, what will be *better?* Often, looking at the obstacles in your path makes them already seem more manageable, especially when considered alongside the benefits of finally doing what needs to be done.

One approach that I recommend is something I call "Let's Make a Deal," after the old television game show. You get to be both Monty Hall and the lucky contestant. You state what has to be done, and you determine how you will tackle it without feeling put upon or out of control. You can offer yourself a small prize: do this job for ten minutes, then take a break and call a friend. And although I never recommend using food as a reward, maybe you *delay* eating dessert one evening after dinner, and make it part of the game: fill one page of your notebook with ideas for your report, and then sit down to enjoy a piece of healthy pie. Very few of us are born perfectly focused or constantly motivated, and I've discovered that success comes from trial and error. Are you someone who responds to pleasurable bribes? Are you the kind of person who hates to tackle a project all alone but is tireless when there's a team or buddy to share the work? Do you tend to procrastinate because you're not sure you're making the right decision, but find it easier to get going once you poll a few good friends to gather support?

Try several different ways of lighting a fire under yourself, and see what feels good. Begin by asking yourself *what you really want.* If what you really want is to get your house painted, even if it means packing up everything you own and living with boxes for a week, you will find a way. And if you can't seem to get started out of fear or insecurity, try to figure out what you need to bolster your confidence—more research? advice from a colleague? This is a great time to dig out and reread the file of congratulatory memos you received the last time you gave a presentation to the marketing department. I remember hearing an old song from World War I that had the doughboys shouting, "We've done it before and we can do it again." You have, and you can!

### A Pearl to Polish

*It's way too easy to focus on your failings, not on your triumphs, especially if you've got a history of being self-critical* (or perhaps a parent or spouse who's tended to pick away at your hard-won self-esteem over the years). Maybe what you need is a kind of "success scrapbook," the kind of thing PR agencies keep to show their clients. Yours doesn't need to be shown to anyone (unless you choose to), but it can be a powerful and encouraging way to chronicle what has made you feel fulfilled over time. A volunteer job that helped your child's school, a fitness accomplishment that surprised even you, visual or written evidence of the healthy changes you've made in your life—these all belong in your "Joy Journal." Practice paging through it when you're feeling shaky or you just want to remember the intense satisfaction you felt on reaching a goal once before.

# Finding a Role Model— and Being One

*To save one life, it is as if you had saved the world.*

—THE TALMUD

$\mathcal{S}$ometimes, when we're trying to change behavior we're not happy with, a role model can make all the difference. From the time I was a child, I learned from my mother and grandmother about caring for the family, about hard work and commitment, and about doing my best. As a businesswoman, I found people to admire on the job who encouraged my ambition to succeed. But when it came to losing weight and keeping it off, I never seemed to find the right model to help me make a real life-change.

Then I reached what for me was a kind of Point of No Return. I was determined to become healthy, to make changes in how I lived and ate so that I wouldn't be a worry or a burden to my children. I taught myself how to cook in a healthy way, and created recipes that would make it possible to continue in my quest week after week. But when it came to making exercise a regular part of my life, I needed help. I needed someone to look up to, someone real. I couldn't hire a personal trainer, and at more than three hundred pounds, I wasn't comfortable with putting on a leotard and trying to do aerobics. But I believed that I could start on my journey to better health by walking. And I took as my role model a woman in my town. Milly was years older than I was, but in much better shape. She walked regularly at the Hart Center, our community health club, and simply by her example and her beautiful, encouraging smile, she helped me get started and keep going. She didn't do it in a big showy way, and not in any kind of public arena, but privately. By her presence, her encouragement, and her kindness, she lifted up my soul.

These days, I walk the country roads near my house, and I ride my bike as often as I can. When we're on the road, I check out the hotel health club, and if I don't manage to fit in a regular-style workout, I walk around the car or mobile home when we gas up. I walk the halls of wherever we're staying. I climb stairs when I can. And I smile at the people who see me pass by, and for a moment, I think of Milly. People have told me that my books and talks have helped them get started on their journeys to better health, and so I feel I am passing on Milly's special legacy. Would it surprise you to know that even if you're many pounds from a weight-loss goal, you might still be someone's role model? It's not about how fit you are, how muscled or young. It's about show-ing up, doing your best, keeping on keeping on, and letting your heart and soul show on the outside. Maybe someone is watching you put one foot in front of the other—someone who needs a spark of hope to take her own first step. Maybe you are providing it without even knowing it. Wouldn't that be a wonderful way to make your world and your community a better place?

Take a moment to think about some of the people who've been your own role models. Some may instantly come to mind, while others may surprise you in a memory. People have always asked me where I found my inspiration in the kitchen, but of course creating recipes isn't all that I love to do. When I was sewing curtains for my new kitchen, I found myself remembering Mrs. Swearingen, my high school home economics teacher. I loved sewing with all my heart, and when the school decided that they would just be offering cooking one year, I was so disappointed. She didn't just sympathize with a student's heartbreak; she put herself on the line for me. She told me that as long as I was willing to come meet with her during her prep hour, and helped her do what needed to be done, she'd help me with my sewing on her own time. To get permission for this special help, she had to go to the principal and the school board. She knew that I wanted to continue learning, and she went the extra mile to help me. With her guidance, I made a beautiful, fully lined coat with bound buttonholes, and a wonderful black silk brocade suit. Mrs. S was every inch the kind of teacher a student dreams of finding. She transformed a girl with basic sewing skills into a real dressmaker, someone who could spread her wings and follow her dreams. A teacher who will give up her own free time to help a student is a special gift, and one whose contribution to your life should be acknowledged.

Of course, finding a sympathetic person to help isn't always easy. I remember when my daughter, Becky, was in high school taking a computer programming language course. She was finding it tough going, and felt if she could just get a little extra help early on, she'd be fine. I suggested she go talk to her teacher, and she got up the courage to ask for his help. Instead of finding a kindred spirit who was happy that one of his students really cared about learning this difficult new subject, he was incredibly rude to her, asking, "Why should I give up my free time just because you're not smart enough to get it in class?" She felt terrible and I felt sad when she told me about his response, because I'd encouraged her to seek his help. But I wanted to show her there was more than one way to get what she needed.

I suggested she look around her class and find someone who was a good student but perhaps shy and open to a new friendship. She chose a young man who today might be called a bit of a "geek," a brilliant but not very popular boy. He agreed to give her some private tutoring, and in two weeks or so, she had it down. For her part, she introduced him to her circle of friends and involved him in some of their activities and parties. He helped her and she helped him, and he was thrilled to do it. It was a real reminder that we are all teachers, and we can help each other if we will only take the time to do it.

(Incidentally, my son Tommy later had Becky's teacher for calculus. When I went to meet with him one evening, he told me that in all his years of teaching he'd seen only a few kids that good in math. Of course I was pleased to hear that, but it also made me burn a little inside. It's easy to teach someone who "gets" it quickly; the real test is helping someone to learn who needs more time to understand!)

When I began losing weight by following healthy, tasty recipes I created myself, I discovered how it felt to be a kind of weight-loss role model, something I'd never figured on being. Everyone looked at my plate and smelled those good aromas and wanted the recipes, but it was more than that. One woman said that if I could do it, then she figured she could too. She started taking care of herself and did really well, and it felt so good to know I'd had a small part in getting her started. Of course, when someone tells you that you're an inspiration, it gives you obligations too. When you become a role model for someone else, you don't want to let him or her down. Maybe you could forget your own goals for a minute, but realizing your visibility makes you more aware of why sticking to your goals is so important.

These days, I get loads of people coming up to me after my speaking engagements who have questions about making a healthy lifestyle work, or about starting a successful business. I've visited with young moms who wanted to start a home business, something they could do while caring for their children. When the conversation turns to goals and dreams, I remind each of them to be true to herself.

I had a long talk with Christie, a thirty-something woman with a husband and two young children at home. She came to me because she wanted to start her own career in publishing. First, I told her, don't forget that I started this when my kids were already raised and out of the house. The years I spent building my business were years of working nights and weekends, time that would have been hard to find if I'd tried this earlier in my life.

It's a question of values for me. I respect ambition and drive, but I also understand what it can take to reach for success. Giving your all to your business may mean letting your family down, so if you decide to pursue a career at the same time you're raising a family, I believe you need to put your family first. It may take longer to reach your goals, but that's better than shortchanging the people you love.

Another woman shared her experiences with me. First, she said, she thought she could be Superwoman, but she realized quite soon that there just weren't enough hours in the day to do what she wanted to do. Eventually, she achieved her dreams of being published, but she did it on a different schedule than she'd originally planned. She wasn't so busy that her kids couldn't talk to her when they needed her.

It's a funny thing about the rosy glow of success: sometimes, in your efforts to be humble and share credit for your accomplishments, you may actually make it all seem easier than it is. By underplaying what it took to get where you did, you may convince people that it all fell in your lap. I always stress the tons of work that Cliff and I did to grow Healthy Exchanges and keep it going. Some people think because you have employees that it doesn't take all that much effort to get the job done. But let me tell you, it takes more than signing the checks to make a business run smoothly over the years. I warn anyone and everyone about to launch a business that they will be surprised by how much work is required beyond what seems obvious. But no matter how well informed and prepared you are up front, you'll discover you haven't thought of everything! The key is to expect the unexpected, don't be ashamed to ask for help when you don't know the answer, and learn from your mistakes—you'll make plenty. We all do.

I always considered Mary Kay Ash a role model of mine, even though we have never met. I read her book, and I listened to her being interviewed on the radio and television, and I always felt that she had her life in order. And her priorities: God first, family second, business third. To me, that's the kind of math that adds up to a good life well lived.

### A Pearl to Polish

*When my friend Milly won first place in her age group (women seventy-plus) at our annual Bix 7-Mile Road Race in Davenport, Iowa, I felt such pride at her accomplishment (especially since the race is run in July, when the heat and humidity are at their highest, and even finishing the race is a badge of honor!). But more than that, I thought about what I might be like when I'm a seventy-year-old lady and still (I hope) lining up for that event. The idea that I would still be fit enough to go the distance made me contemplate my own later years with optimism and a positive attitude about aging. I'd found a role model who could inspire me now and for years to come. Why not make a list of the people who make you feel optimistic and hopeful about your own future? At the same time, take a look around and see if there's someone you could "lift up" by your example. Finding a role model and being one are both wonderful goals!*

# Don't Be in a Hurry . . .

*I have learned this at least by my experiment: if one advances confidently in the direction of his dreams, and endeavors to live the life he has imagined, he will meet with a success unexpected in common hours.*

—HENRY DAVID THOREAU

*W*henever people hear the story of my 130-pound weight loss, they almost always want to know how long it took. It's often the first question anyone is asked about success in losing weight, but I'd love to see that change once and for all!

It's such a "dieting" question, and hidden in that question is a desire to judge how well the program or the secret "works." Can I lose ten pounds in two weeks? Say the answer is yes, you can. *Okay, I can survive anything for two weeks.* Will I carve off twenty pounds before my daughter's wedding in May? If it sounds doable, then sure, *I'll get acupuncture or take injections of some mysterious concoctions or live on liquids that taste so awful going down that you have to follow them with a Diet Coke chaser.*

Each time people ask that question about the time it took to lose the weight, I want to take them under my wing and suggest they're asking the wrong question. In fact, they've been asking the wrong question all their lives, which is why they're still haunted by their failure to get to and remain at a healthy body weight.

There is nothing much any of us can do about the passage of time. We can use cosmetics to disguise the physical evidence of aging, we can dress youthfully, exercise for health, drink moderately, take vitamins—and still the clock runs away with our lives. On Monday, the week may seem endlessly long, but when Sunday arrives, you wonder how a week could have passed so quickly!

And yet, when it comes to choosing a program to lose weight, too few people ask themselves, "Can I eat this way for the rest of my life and not feel deprived? Can I enjoy food instead of hiding in my house to avoid having to face all that temptation in the world? Can I eat meals with my family, celebrate joyful occasions, dine on pie and potatoes, and not die of guilt?"

Instead, they want to know how long it will take, how long until they can stop doing what they're willing to do to *lose* the weight. And built into that way of thinking is disaster, because it will never be enough just to lose the weight and go back to old eating habits. It will never last. So no matter how fast it falls off your body, it won't stay off.

When I tell people not to be in a hurry to get the pounds off, I speak from experience—mine, and that of so many other people who have finally understood that this kind of life success can't be measured in weeks or even months. I know it requires a complete turnabout for most of the people who hear me say that, because a time frame seems to give a kind of hope, especially to those who've struggled at a particular point for a long time.

But promising results that are linked to a specific duration of time is a kind of lie, so I don't do it. Neither, thank heavens, do the better weight-loss support group organizations—at least, not anymore. It's harder to sell people on a book or a video or meetings without making those kinds of promises, but it's an honest approach, and that's why now it's actually part of a consumer protection law.

Why else do people want to know how long it will take?

For some, it's a fear of losing motivation, since their past experience tells them that motivation, that mysterious force that keeps you on track, lasts only so long—and then it vanishes. "I'm feeling really motivated right now," one woman told me not long ago. "I've got my high school reunion coming up in three months, so I'm determined to stick with it." Yes, she was very determined, but only convinced that she'd stay that way until the last member of the class of '75 left the building!

"What about after the reunion?" I asked gently. "What about all those months and years to come? Wouldn't you like to feel as good as you can for as long as possible?" She nodded, but she looked doubtful that such a thing was really possible.

Others need to know "how long?" because they're sure that boredom will set in. Boredom with what you're eating or how you're getting your exercise is often the speedy death of "motivation." I remember overhearing a group of people discussing how bored they were on the high-protein diet they'd been following for a few weeks. "At the beginning," one man said, "I was so thrilled I could have bacon and eggs every morning and not worry about gaining weight. But now, oh now would I ever kill for a big fresh fruit salad!" The others agreed, and a woman added, "Well, I'm going to do this for just one more month, and then I'm taking a vacation from anything that looks like a diet."

Uh-oh.

She's so tired of the way she's eating that she's planning to eat everything in sight! I'm not an "I-told-you-so" sort of person, but I fear that whatever weight she's managed to lose up to that point may very likely return with a vengeance. And the cycle will begin again. It's such an unhappy one, but it's not the only option you've got.

Let's start with an entirely different premise. Suppose you'd been selected for a secret government research project, and you were going to live in a remote area for the next two years. (Not unlike the Biosphere people, I know.) As part of your preparation, you were asked to list the foods you liked to eat, because someone had to stock the pantry and freezer for you. No one is making any value judgments about what's on your list—they just want you to be happy while you're stuck in that underground laboratory. Suppose you began by listing your favorite foods: cherry pie, tacos, corn chowder, chicken à la king, macaroni and cheese, coleslaw and potato salad . . . You get the idea. Now, remember, no one is telling you not to eat what you enjoy, right? So you can be honest, and you get to have the dishes you love best. Isn't that a recipe for long-term satisfaction?

You could never eat that way on a crash diet!

That's why people keep falling off the wagon and regaining whatever they've managed to lose during a period of deprivation.

This is kind of like the task I set for myself when I created my first Healthy Exchanges recipes. I decided to be an experiment of one (I could say two, since I was also feeding Cliff, but since he wasn't specifically focused on losing weight and regaining health at the time, I considered him to be "coming along for the ride"). I realized that there wasn't any way I could survive the next two years of my life, in an underground lab or in DeWitt, Iowa, without getting to eat the kinds of foods I liked. So I decided to become a kitchen chemist, mixing and fixing all kinds of foods until I found healthy ways to prepare the dishes I enjoyed.

What I discovered, besides a passion for creating recipes that now number in the thousands, was that *it could be done.*

I could eat what I liked, I could lose weight and keep it off, and as time passed, I didn't grow bored or bitter. I didn't lose motivation because I didn't need nearly as much as I feared. I was just living each day, eating healthily, exercising moderately, and keeping a positive attitude that helped me set goals, reach them, and set some more!

I haven't banned the calendar or the clock from my house. But I no longer count the days and weeks and months that I'm eating this way. Well, I do celebrate each year of healthy living and continued success, but the rest of the time, I'm not wondering how long it will last, I'm not worrying whether I'll grow bored, and I'm not in a hurry to "get there."

It turned out that "there" was a place I already was, that while a goal weight is a great destination to reach, it's not the only purpose of the journey. When you're enjoying your life, as most of us do when we're on vacation, you look out the window, you smile as the scenery passes, you even slow down here and there to relish the view and take pleasure in each new experience.

*You're not in a hurry for it to end.* You're delighting in each minute of the trip. That's how I want to feel as I move through my life. And as unfamiliar as it may be to make that philosophy part of your commitment to your healthy lifestyle, it's how you want to feel, too.

Now, I'm not suggesting that we stop getting on the scale once a week to see how it's going. (Besides, I know you'd be way too tempted to give that up!) But maybe the next time someone asks you how much weight you've lost, and you say the number, if the follow-up question is, "And how long did it take you?" you decide not to answer with the number of weeks or months or years. Instead, why not smile confidently and say, "I don't exactly remember when I started, but I'm enjoying the journey and I feel good about how far I've come."

I think this is a great notion for anyone who's frustrated with a slow weight loss, or who's been facing a "stuck" needle on the scale for a few weeks. I know one woman who deliberately takes off her watch (which is one of those digital ones with the date on it) before she gets on the scale, just to remind herself that she's not counting the time it takes to lose her weight. (I asked her if she knew how much the watch weighed, concerned that she was also doing it to save a few ounces. When she told me she didn't know, I was glad to hear it!)

If enough of us start refusing to measure our weight loss in weeks, maybe it'll launch a trend away from that "hurry-up" mentality that dooms so many eager dieters. Even when we tell ourselves that we're willing to eat this way for the rest of our lives, it can take awhile to believe it deep down. But keep trying, because it's amazingly liberating to stop measuring how long it takes, and to start making every day count, no matter what the scale says.

### A Pearl to Polish

*What did you do yesterday with those twenty-four precious hours? Did you waste any of them feeling guilty about the food you ate or didn't eat? Did you lose track of any of them because you were worrying about your appearance or weighed down by a dozen new books that promised to get the weight off faster than what you're already doing? Did you spend any of your waking hours just breathing deeply and feeling good about your accomplishments as a human being? Learn from the past, then put it away, and live, really live, for today.*

# Counting Your Blessings

---

*When one door of happiness closes, another opens; but often we look so long at the closed door that we do not see the one which has opened for us.*

—HELEN KELLER

*W*ith only a few days to go until Cliff's and my anniversary, I've been thinking even more than usual about counting my blessings and giving thanks. I've never been one of those people who saves up her thanks for just one day in the year. Rather, I'm a believer in expressing gratitude every day.

I try not to let a day go by without thanking God for His many gifts, not the least of which has been the opportunity to share my common-folk healthy recipes and my commonsense approach to healthy living. It's been a magnificent mission so far, one that has transformed my life in so many ways, I can't begin to count them. So I make sure to thank the Lord for the big things—the talent to create, the courage to share my message, and the strength to keep up my busy schedule week after week and year after year. I thank Him for sending me Cliff, such a perfect partner in work and in life, a man who has been by my side in everything for more than twenty years now. And of course I thank Him for the never-ending blessings of my children and grandchildren, who are such an important part of my life.

But I also thank Him for an amazing variety of little things—the glorious colors of fall foliage I drink in as I ride my bike along a country road; the sweet flavor of ripe strawberries sliced into a summer salad; the joyful song of a passing bird that fills my heart with happiness. I give thanks because in the moment that I express my gratitude for the big and the little things I am blessed to have in my life, I experience a kind of grace, a moment of connection with what is eternal.

Saying thank you, silently or aloud, seated in a church or pedaling along the perimeter of our property, is how I acknowledge the powerful role that spirit plays in my daily existence. In the midst of all the clutter of my desk and the many interruptions throughout my day, those moments stand out in sharp contrast—and they add so much to the quality of my life. And while the media shines the brightest light on the subject around the fourth Thursday in November, I want to encourage you to make counting your blessings as close to a daily observance as you can.

Since I'm such an early bird, starting my days by collecting my thoughts on the subject seems to work best for me. It's quiet in the house, and since I wake up remarkably clearheaded, I feel ready to reflect on the preceding day and night. I don't have a particular ritual or standard way of focusing on the subject, but each of us finds our own best way. I remember reading an article not long ago that suggested keeping a journal of gratitude, a place to record each day or evening what you are most grateful for right at that time. I think it's a lovely idea, and one from which many people may draw strength. On those days when your life seems most chaotic and you're struggling with negativity, paging through your notes of thanks for what is good in your life can help steady your resolve to "hang in there"!

For some, those quiet minutes before you turn out the light and go to sleep may be the perfect time to count your blessings and give thanks. It's always been a traditional time to make spiritual connections, even since childhood, when you learned "Now I lay me down to sleep . . ." and whispered to God to bless Mommy and Daddy and all of your loved ones. Collecting your thoughts at night may also help you put your mind at rest, so that your sleep is peaceful and your body truly refreshed when you awaken in the morning.

The timing is up to you, and after a few days or weeks of regular reflection, you'll likely find out what works best for you. What's important is to make time for this communion of spirit, this chance to put aside daily cares and struggles, and to listen to your heart.

One of the ways I use the quiet time in the morning to get in touch with my own soul is sitting at my desk and reading through the many e-mails and letters I receive on a daily basis. I've been blessed to have so many people share their lives with me through correspondence, and hearing how they've transformed their lives through making a commitment to live healthier blesses me as it has clearly blessed them.

When I created the HELP Success Story contest in my newsletter, I expected to receive entries that celebrated satisfying weight losses, letters that trumpeted great improvement on cholesterol counts and blood sugar levels, as well as mail that described a variety of workouts that had truly worked for people. But the thread running through most of the entries was how these lifestyle changes had transformed the rest of the writer's life in so many ways. One of the winners I chose had counted her blessings, big and small, and wanted to share what she'd learned with the rest of my Healthy Exchanges family members.

Jill wrote, "I can't believe how much better I feel all around. I have so much more energy now—I can't believe I'm even the same person anymore! I am much more active with my children (aged seven and three) and it feels wonderful! My cholesterol level is down to 170, which my doctor says is EXCELLENT. I serve much more nutritious and balanced meals to my family, and with all this extra energy, I have become more organized in many areas of my life." Her family had been thrilled by the changes in her, but Jill recognized that some of the changes were more subtle: "Even my asthma seems to have decreased in severity. And probably one of the most important changes is that for the first time in years, I am happy with my body. I'm sure I will never be model-thin (don't think I'd want to be), but I realize that being fit and healthy and feeling great is so much more important than a number on the scale or a dress size. By the way,

I now wear a size 10, which is what I wore in my 'thin days' in high school!"

For Jill, counting her blessings was more important than counting each quarter pound lost on the scale. Yes, she succeeded in reaching a weight-loss goal through her lifestyle changes, but by focusing on the many ways that her life had been blessed in the process, she stayed grounded in what was truly important: living each day to the fullest and doing her best.

Maybe you are going through troubling times right now, and counting your blessings is as far away from your thoughts as Mars is from Earth! Don't browbeat yourself about it, because that kind of negativity just makes it harder to take good care of yourself and those you love. If the difficulties you're facing over-shadow the good in your life at this moment, take comfort in knowing that you can begin to change that with this one exercise. Even if you have to lock yourself in the bathroom for ten min-utes to find a moment of peace and quiet, do it—just this once, and it will start to get easier. Take a pad, and if you haven't got a pad, use the back of an envelope or a piece of junk mail. Grab a pen or pencil or one of your kids' crayons if that's all you can find, and make a little list of your blessings. I'd like you to try for three items the first time out, but feel free to list as many as you can. Don't skip the little things, as they can add up to an aston-ishing amount of joy.

What's your favorite thing about yourself? Start with that. Your great green eyes, your wacky sense of humor, your curly brown hair, your voice rising in song in your church choir . . . they're all blessings, and they're all yours. Okay, what else? Think of your family and friends, and write down one or two of the ways those relationships have blessed you, today or recently. Did your sister make you laugh on the phone this morning? Did your new neighbors invite you for dinner next week? Did your boss praise you for something you worked hard on and finished on time? It all counts.

Now let's focus on a way in which you blessed yourself today. Did you squeeze in a fifteen-minute walk during your lunch hour instead of gobbling fast food at your desk? (No points deducted if you splurged on a new lipstick on your excursion, either—it made you feel good!) Did you stock your fridge with healthy snacks for when you come home from work exhausted, and did you enjoy every bite of the one you chose today? Good work!

Try to think of something you learned or did in the past twenty-four hours that can help you change your life for the better. Did you read and then tear out a healthy recipe from the newspaper and plan to prepare it this weekend? Did you watch a program on TV that encouraged women to lift weights to avoid osteoporosis, and did you then retrieve your set of dumbbells from under the bed so you could use them a couple of times this week? Did you receive a compliment on your appearance today, and instead of saying, "This old thing?" did you catch yourself and remember to answer, "Thank you"?

You *are* blessed, then. Blessed by your intelligence and willingness to change. Blessed by an open mind that refuses to give up even when you feel discouraged. Blessed by more strength than you knew you had. But as you start to "keep score" of the big and little ways in which you are blessed and in which you bless yourself, you'll discover that taking a few minutes to count your blessings is time well spent indeed.

## *A Pearl to Polish*

*Too many of us don't make time to express gratitude—to God, to those we love and who love us, and even to praise ourselves. But it's never too late to start. Why not stop counting pounds, inches, and what you've got in the bank, and start counting your blessings today?*

# Find the Heart
# to Begin

*Begin; to begin is half the work. Let half still remain; again begin this, and thou wilt have finished.*

—AUSONIUS, LATIN POET

*H*ow do you know when it's the right time to make a change in your life?

*Is* there such a time?

So often you feel unhappy about where you are, but you also feel overwhelmed and uncertain about how to stop feeling stuck and move on. Whatever emotion has you in its grip—fear, anger, guilt, helplessness, hopelessness, even disgust—can be strong enough to discourage you from taking action.

I remember in those years when I was feeling desperate about my weight problem, I told myself I was willing to suffer just about anything for a speedy result—starvation, injections, pills, whatever promised to deliver instant change.

It took me a lot of years to accept the truth that there is no such thing as instant change. There's no magic or secret, just commitment and hard work, along with my daily prayer, "Please, God, help me help myself just for today."

Still, when people call or write to me about their own problems, I know that many of them are hoping for a quick fix, an easy answer. Just as I did, they're wishing for something that doesn't exist. What they want and need means digging deeper, finding the heart of the problem and beginning the healing process.

A woman called me one night recently, overcome by feelings of frustration and worthlessness. She had recently given up smoking and had gained a lot of weight. Her husband had been extremely critical of her, increasing her pain and feelings of isolation. "Maybe he thinks he's helping me by pointing it out," she said. "But he's not telling me anything I don't already know, and it hurts."

As we talked quietly, I could hear the exhaustion in her voice as well as her fear that nothing would help. I responded to that first of all.

"You're already doing something about the problem by sharing it," I told her. "Give yourself credit for that. You've also accomplished something really difficult in deciding to quit smoking. Do you know how much strength it takes to give up a real physical addiction like that?"

She seemed surprised at my words. She hadn't felt good about herself in so long, she never expected anyone to acknowledge her in this way. It gave her permission to admit it to herself, and to pat herself on the back just a little.

We talked about how she'd replaced her oral fix with food, so that food had become her enemy, her prison. Because of her weight gain, she rarely left the house, and when she did, she wore the one outfit that fit and felt comfortable, a pair of old sweats. Every time she looked in the mirror, she felt defeated before she could even begin. But she told me she wasn't willing to live this way anymore.

*Those are the words I want to hear.*

In fact, saying them out loud just as the character in the movie *Network* did, that you're not going to take it anymore, is one of the first steps on the path to making a change in your life.

I want to give my help to people who are willing to work, and willing to change. Turning your problems over to a Higher Being, acknowledging your imperfections and asking for help is a start. But don't expect your problem to be solved by God. When you "turn over" your problems, you're simply asking for guidance, just as when you were a child you turned your scraped knees and hurt feelings over to your parents. But even a child who's comforted and advised how to take care still has to make the choices: to play safely, to fight or not with another child.

The woman, whom I'll call Maryanne, came to me looking for advice about her weight problem. But the help she needed involved much more than what to eat and when to eat it. I wanted to help her make different choices, choices that would help her take control of her life. Sometimes we don't make the right choices—after all, we're all human. But help is still there if we're willing to look for it.

Remember the Bible verse "I look up into the hills from whence cometh my help"? Take a moment to think: Where does *your* help come from? I pray to God, but I know that the help I need doesn't come from Him alone. Some comes from my family; some from my friends; and some from looking deep into my own heart.

Maryanne didn't ask me how long it would take her to get the weight off; she knew instinctively that it was only part of the problem. Her expectations were realistic; she recognized, as many people don't, that you can't go from A to Z in one giant step. Instead, you usually need to work on a number of small things.

I like to say, "Focus on what you *can* do, not on what seems impossible." Maybe it'll help to think of your life as a messy room. You open the door and you want to scream, it's such a disaster area. Already you feel exhausted at the idea of cleaning it up and putting everything away.

STOP. Close your eyes. Now, open them again and choose three things nearest at hand. Pick them up and walk out of the room. That's how you're going to begin. Then when you come back there's less to do. Start by making order in one little corner of the room, then move on to the next. Eventually you will be able to see that you're making progress, but I ask you to keep going even when it seems as if little progress has been made. And remember that what matters is *your* view of things, not someone else's. *You* can see that you've tidied the room (or your life) partway, even though someone else can't.

Recognize that you can't do too many things at once. Sure,

you can nibble away at more than one thing, but don't overdo it. Don't do too much, but don't accept too little either.

For Maryanne, we identified each of several problems related to the bigger one, and decided how she could cope with it.

First, oral gratification. Her mouth was missing some satisfaction because she'd given up her post-meal cigarette. I suggested she plan to enjoy a low-fat, low-sugar *crunchy* dessert from one of my cookbooks every single night for a week. I wasn't asking her to deny the desire, just to *plan* for it.

Second, to help her remind herself she was finished eating, we devised a simple behavior change: after the final bite, she would crumple her napkin and put it on her plate. I asked her to do it even if she felt a little silly, because it would be a clear, visual reminder of her choice to stop.

Third, she needed to get out of the house, both because exercise would help her burn calories and because staying in the house kept her close to the kitchen, where she was doing most of her overeating. Even though she has a young baby at home, I told her to put the baby in the stroller and walk to the park. It's good advice for anyone stuck in a rut at home. Walk around the block if there's no park, and if the weather's bad, walk around the mall. If there's no mall, try any large store except a supermarket! But walk. Just walk.

Next, I suggested she work a little on making herself feel better about her appearance. How? Perhaps by buying herself one pair of slacks that fit, and one attractive top that fits her well *now*. I always say, dress for now. You've got to look good for yourself *today* before you can look good tomorrow. Don't wait until you're the perfect size to take care of yourself. Put on a nice pair of ear-rings; take a moment to put on lipstick. It's a positive approach to living in the moment.

But while it's important to look as good for yourself as you can, what's more important is caring about what's inside you. Ask yourself what was important to you before you began feeling bad about yourself. Get in touch with those feelings—and acknowl-edge them in the most positive way you can. Remember you are the same person you always were. Don't allow external things to pick away at your self-esteem until you feel worthless. You're no less a person than you were before. You may be even better be-cause you've survived.

Last, and maybe most important, I asked her to take a pad and each day write down at least three things for which she de-served praise, including any of those listed above. I wanted her to spend a couple of minutes every day thinking good thoughts about herself, reminding herself that she had done something positive for herself.

But this Positive Attitude diary isn't about either/or, or about perfection. If the only choice is smoking three packs a day or going cold turkey, for example, you may find yourself unable to quit or doomed to repeated failures. That's what my life was like as a professional dieter. I had to be perfect, or else I fell off the wagon, unable to climb back on.

Instead, this is about doing your best each day, and if you make a mistake, *you go on.* Give yourself credit: every time you park your car and walk a couple of extra blocks is a drop in the bucket to get-ting more fit. Every pat on the back you give yourself helps you build healthy self-esteem. And if you plan to eat one cookie and instead you eat three, but *then* you stop, you've *still* accomplished something. In the old days you might have finished the bag.

These are just a few baby steps, but each one can have a powerful impact on how you feel about yourself. Think of those steps as movement forward, movement away from what isn't working, movement toward the goal you want to achieve.

You'll feel better when you're moving. It's almost a kind of symbol that you're doing something positive—and your body is coming along for the ride. Sitting or standing still, you can't change where you are or where you're going. It takes moving forward to get somewhere new.

I never studied physics, but a friend once explained to me that there's a principle that says: A body at rest stays at rest. A body in motion stays in motion. What does that mean? Well, it's easier to keep an object moving once it's moving, but it takes major effort to get it started. That's what you're feeling when it feels so hard to take that first step. But if you can get yourself in motion, mentally, physically, and emotionally, acknowledging that you have the power to move from point A to point B, you'll find it much easier to keep going.

Remember when you were learning to walk? First you could only crawl. Then one day you stood up, and before too much longer you managed to walk a few shaky steps to Mama. You may not really remember how good it felt to do that, but try—and then recognize the parallel in your life now. Take the little step or two. Cheer yourself. Tomorrow, take a few more. Eventually you'll be walking, then maybe even a jog. Then you can go anywhere you dream.

There's no way to begin but to begin. Begin today.

### A Pearl to Polish

*God responds when you act. When you move in the right direction, you may feel His hand giving you a gentle push forward.*

# Handling Difficult People and the Obstacle Course of Life

*Life's ups and downs provide windows of opportunity to determine your values and goals. Think of using all obstacles as stepping stones to build the life you want.*

—MARSHA SINETAR, AUTHOR

*D*o you ever find yourself saying, "I could stick to a healthy eating plan if I didn't have to cook for my meat-and-potatoes husband and my three picky kids"? Or perhaps, "Nothing tempts me too much in everyday life, but I've got three weddings in the next six weeks, and I'll have to eat whatever they serve, which means dieting disaster!" Or maybe, "I was doing so well on my program, cooking healthy dishes and making time for exercise, until I had to go home for the holidays. All that family pressure, not to mention being surrounded by cake, cookies, and candy—I ate everything that wasn't nailed down!"

Life is a kind of obstacle course, isn't it? Just when the road ahead appears smooth, you've got difficult people to contend with, special occasions to confront, stress at month's end and the beginning of each new year. You can try to surround yourself with positive people who support you in your effort to live healthy, but whoops, there comes an unexpected "saboteur" from the shadows—and you discover you're still susceptible to emotional binges or attacks of low self-esteem!

It would be terrific if you could select just which people and events would be part of your life, but that's not an option for most of us. We can make some decisions about the ways our lives unfold, but we don't control everything that happens to us.

**All we can control is how we react to it.**

Turning a negative situation into a positive one takes preparation, practice, and a willingness to make mistakes—and learn from them. But first you need to recognize who's doing what, before you can decide how to handle what life tosses in your path.

Let's start with the people who make life difficult:

The **Saboteurs** compliment you on your weight loss, congratulate you on getting your cholesterol under control, smile when you share your positive report from your cardiologist. Then they serve only high-fat foods when they invite you for dinner or present you with a five-pound box of chocolate truffles on your birthday. They'd swear that they're on your side, that they have your best interests at heart, but consciously or unconsciously, they're trying to sabotage your good efforts.

Why would anyone do this? Well, they may be jealous of your success. They may simply be thoughtless when it comes to choosing dinner recipes or a festive gift. They may want company in a lifestyle that is sedentary and unhealthy. ("You were more fun when you were heavier and liked to go out drinking Friday nights," someone might say when confronted.)

Sometimes saboteurs are very close to home and don't realize what they're doing. Perhaps your grandmother loves to bake for her grandkids, and she uses her rich desserts to show how much she loves you. Is she truly a saboteur? In a way, she is, because she's offering you food you don't want, and saying no can be difficult because of the emotional ties you feel. But loving her doesn't mean you have to go along with the "sabotage." You can tell her you're full but would love to take a piece home. You can ooh and aah over a small piece, then quickly discard the rest when no one is looking. You can promise her you'll have a piece later, and add, "It looks scrumptious!" That way, she gets appreciation, you get a sense of being in control of your food choices, and love finds a way.

What other techniques work with saboteurs? If you're dealing with a true friend, get the issue right out in the open. Say, "You're a wonderful cook, but my doctor warned me about keeping my cholesterol down. The next time you invite me for brunch, could we skip the quiche and maybe have some of your luscious pancakes or French toast?" You're asking for help nicely, you're offering options that provide a "win-win" situation for both of you, and you're showing that you value the friendship enough to be honest.

However, if your saboteur isn't receptive to your needs, you may have to decide to limit the amount of time you spend together. Or make a date for a movie or shopping that takes the focus away from food. And if someone keeps giving you inappropriate food gifts, just say thanks and pass them along to a senior center or nursing home.

How about a group of difficult people I call **Naysayers** and **Discouragers**?

These are the people who try to talk you out of what you've chosen to do, who downplay your successes and criticize your efforts. Even if you've lost twenty-five pounds by following the HELP plan, for example, these people may pressure you to give up what's working for you and take their advice instead. "You can't lose weight unless you cut down on carbohydrates," someone may insist. "No white bread or pasta," another says firmly. Still another snickers at your exercise program, which consists of a brisk daily walk around the neighborhood. "If you're not lifting weights, you'll never get anywhere," she says. "If you're not sweating up a storm, you're not doing your heart any good," another vows.

*Aaaargh!*

No matter what you're doing, it seems, someone in your life knows better.

No matter how good you feel or how healthy you're getting, someone is convinced that your program needs tweaking, that your doctor doesn't know what he's talking about, that your dietitian hasn't read the latest research. They only seem happy when they've managed to make you doubt yourself and everything you believe in. No matter what you've accomplished, they announce that you could have done much better, lost weight faster, saved money, whatever—if only you'd done it *their way.*

My response to the naysayers: Say nay! No! No thank you! Thanks for your suggestions, but I'm happy with how things are.

Or if you aren't comfortable saying "No" right off, simply say, "Thanks—I'll definitely give it some thought." Oscar Wilde once commented that the only thing to do with good advice is to "pass it on. It is never any good to oneself."

We live in a world where the next great thing is always just around the corner. The perfect and easy diet plan. The amazing time-saving exercise program. A better job, a richer boyfriend, your chance to win a multimillion-dollar payoff in a sweepstakes. All of us are bombarded with encouragement to change what we're doing and seize the moment—buy the hot Internet stock, bet on the winning horse, invent a better mousetrap!

I'd be the last person to try to talk you out of pursuing your dreams and ambitions. That's not at all what I mean. But I've observed that many people struggling with health problems and weight issues are vulnerable to naysayers and discouragers, who often take the form of people trying to sell you false hopes. Late-night television is crammed with infomercials offering speedy weight loss in four easy payments, fitness programs that help you shape up while you sleep, quick-fix financial programs with no money down—all designed to enrich their creators while bankrupting you—financially *and* emotionally.

How can you cope with the naysayers and discouragers in your life? What should you say to your mother-in-law, who tells you that your skin is going to sag now that you've lost weight? What about the colleague at work who asks you (as one of mine did me some years ago), "How long do you think you'll keep the weight off this time?" Those seeds of self-doubt don't require much encouragement to grow and strangle your hard-won hope and self-esteem!

This is where I think practice comes in. It may make you feel foolish to stand in front of the mirror and practice responses to such remarks, but actually forming the words and saying them aloud will make it easier when you're challenged by someone in real time. The point is not to get into long-winded arguments, which generally end with both parties feeling angry or hurt. Instead, you want to roll with the punches you receive, answer lightly but confidently, and *move on.* Tell your mother-in-law that you've discovered a marvelous toning exercise for your facial muscles, and you'll make a photocopy for her if she'd like. Or say, "My doctor says my skin is still young enough to tighten up and look wonderful. Phew, what a relief!" Smile at your colleague and say, "Well, I'm not psychic and I can't foretell the future, but I'm really happy with how I feel now." Or try, "I'm in this for the long run. Who wouldn't be, when I look and feel this good?" Add, "I feel lucky to have found a healthy lifestyle I can live with from now on. Here, try these amazing brownies!"

By meeting negative comments with a positive attitude, you transform a difficult moment into a winning one. It may not be easy the first few times, but you'll get better with practice.

Another group of difficult people I want to mention are those I call **Energy Zappers.** You know the ones I mean: the friend who promises to meet you for a walk before work but then doesn't show up; the sister who invites you to go shopping but then can't settle on a store; the buddy at work who keeps asking you to lunch and then spends the entire hour complaining about work. These individuals aren't as obviously difficult as the other types, but all the same, they can exhaust you, steal your momentum, create a mood of negativity that colors your entire day.

It can be tricky to figure out how to cope with the drain on your positive energy. You want to spend time with your sister; you were hoping to get your friend to be more active; you're new in the office and had hoped this person might help you get acclimated. Instead, spending time with these people has the power to drag you down.

Don't let it! The best way to handle an energy zapper is with gentle control. Tell your friend you're going to call her ten minutes before you're supposed to meet, because you really want to see her. Tell your sister that you need to visit two specific stores, then ask her when you make the date what she wants to accomplish that day. Tell your officemate (after you've patiently listed to five or ten minutes of her moans and groans) that you're sorry to hear how frustrated she is, but maybe together you two can institute some changes in the workplace. Create an alliance with your energy "enemy" and you're more than likely to prevent a fight or disagreement. Instead of feeling powerless and going along with what you don't want to do, seize the day—and give yourself a pat on the back.

Sometimes, of course, what causes the greatest stress in our lives is a change in our daily schedules—planned or unplanned. Just when you thought you had life under control (or at least the happy illusion of it!), your baby-sitter calls in sick, your boss asks you to work late, or your mother volunteers your help for a charity auction. Your plan for the day, the week, or the month gets shaken up—and you need to recover fast.

Maybe the disruption in your schedule is a pleasant one but still produces a stress reaction. Your husband surprises you with a weekend at a country inn, your boss informs you that you've been promoted and will be attending a national convention next month, your best friend from college calls to say she's getting married and wants you to be a bridesmaid. In a moment, your life becomes more complicated and you have to figure out how to handle the hurdles in your path.

You love the idea of a romantic weekend—in principle, anyway. But you've got four loads of laundry you'd planned to do Saturday morning, and you'd made plans with a friend to meet at the Y for a workout in the afternoon. You're supposed to rehearse with the church choir Sunday morning, and oh yes, you'd promised your boss you'd proofread the company newsletter over the weekend. Instead of feeling excited and relaxed, you're stressed-out—and ready to reach for the nearest box of cookies!

These bumps in the road do keep life interesting, but they also require a willingness to be flexible and a readiness to cope with unexpected changes. The person you used to be (before you chose to tackle life with a positive attitude, of course) might have reacted by bingeing on fast food while you washed and folded clothes into the wee hours of the morning. You might have wallowed in guilt over missing the choir rehearsal and perhaps even waited until the last minute to cancel plans for the gym. The weekend away would have filled you with fears about what you were going to do or where you'd be eating.

But now that you've decided to revel in life's unpredictability, to make the most of what comes your way, you can cope with a renewed confidence. You call your friend and the choir director, make your apologies, promise to reschedule the gym for a weeknight and to practice on your own with a music cassette, then turn to the practical problems of escaping for a weekend. You sort through the laundry, postpone the sheets and towels because you've got plenty in the linen closet, do two loads Friday evening, and ask your family to help put the folded clothes away. You decide to bring a copy of the newsletter to look over if and when your husband takes a nap, but you also know that you will have time in the office Monday morning to finish checking it.

Problems listed, coped with, settled. Now—off for a well-deserved weekend!

But wait! What about the food? Will you be able to find something healthy to eat on the menu? What if everything is covered in cream sauce? What if—

You've learned to ask for what you need, and there isn't a restaurant kitchen in the world that won't be responsive when a customer has health requirements related to food. Yes, you could check the inn's website for a copy of their dinner menu, or you could call ahead and ask about dining options in the area. But you'll be fine walking into the unknown, the same as you would be walking into any restaurant and ordering what you want to eat. That's what all your months of practice have produced: a confident person who isn't afraid to make decisions about what to have for dinner!

The same holds true when it comes to representing your company at the conference. Start with the practical issues: clear your calendar for the convention dates, arrange a cash advance for expenses, discuss with your boss which clients you should invite to dinner, research the best restaurants, make reservations, and so on. Do you have a choice of hotels? Check to see which one is most convenient to the convention center, and which one has a health club or pool. When you schedule appointments, try to set aside time for yourself; when you select restaurants, choose those that offer a variety of healthy choices. You're not helpless in the face of the unknown; you have the experience and the tools to cope with just about anything. (Except, perhaps, a really unattractive bridesmaid's dress! But let's be optimistic that your friend will chooses a color and style that will help make you look and feel great!)

I chose the image of an obstacle course for this chapter for several reasons: first, running a real one requires all different kinds of skills—running, jumping, climbing, swinging on ropes, and scaling walls. Well, life also requires that we have a variety of skills for coping, and the more confident we are in our preparation, the better we handle the stresses we face.

But running an obstacle course isn't something we're born to do. And doing it well takes training, skill, a certain amount of agility, and a willingness to keep trying even when we're struggling to clear a particular obstruction. So, too, does life demand that we tackle what's hard, that we practice our skills until we feel we can move forward with assurance. On some days, you may not be convinced you've got what it takes, but if you're determined to give it your best shot, you'll get there eventually.

### A Pearl to Polish

*With experience and with time, handling difficult people and unexpected bumps on the road to health gets easier. Give yourself time to get it right, and celebrate each experience that builds your stamina and ability to cope. You might decide to keep an Obstacle Course Diary, reviewing how you faced difficult people and challenging decisions. Over time, you'll see evidence of how much you've grown.*

# No More Being a Victim!

*Never tell me the odds!*
— HAN SOLO, IN *THE EMPIRE STRIKES BACK*

$\mathcal{W}$hen something doesn't go as planned, do you find yourself saying, "It always happens to me. The doctor keeps me waiting. The paperboy throws the paper in the wet grass. The restaurant runs out of what I wanted for dessert. The library doesn't have the book I want. I'm always in the slowest checkout line. I never order the right thing. Nothing I do turns out right. I'm just not lucky—"

Sound familiar?

It's old "poor, pitiful me," rearing her curly head! And even if your plaintive wails momentarily garner sympathy from those around you, the image you project is one of powerlessness. You're helpless in the face of adversity, you're unable to get what you want or succeed in what you're attempting because the odds are stacked against you. You're not in control of your life, and what's more, you never were.

Why?

Because you see yourself as a *victim.*

A victim doesn't have to take any responsibility for what goes wrong, because she or he is simply being buffeted by outside forces. Someone else is pulling the strings, directing the play that is your life.

That kind of passive acceptance can easily become a way of life. Before you know it, the messages you've sent your brain create what is known as a self-fulfilling principle: you expect life to send you lemons, so that is all you ever seem to get, and because your pitcher has a crack in it and you're out of Sweet 'n Low, you never, ever make lemonade.

For many people, these kind of defeated announcements, these demands for sympathy, are spoken unconsciously, without any real awareness that you're setting yourself up to suffer and fail. Most of them have even become clichés. They're like verbal shrugs of the shoulders. "Oh, woe is me," as they used to say in olden times, and truer words were never spoken. You actually become what you say, identifying yourself as the thing you most fear and deny.

Here's the problem: When you keep announcing your victimhood, when you beat yourself over the head with phrases like, "Oh, it's all my fault," or "I never know what to do," you create an environment for failure and disappointment to flourish.

Identifying with the victim mentality is a problem in all kinds of areas, but it's particularly troubling when you're struggling to lose weight or desperate to improve your health. Have you ever found yourself saying, "Oh, diets don't work for me," or "Exercise is boring"? Have you shaken your head and muttered, "No matter what I eat, I can't lose weight"? Yes, I know these are only words, but your brain hears them and believes. By taking on the role of the victim, you set yourself up for failure.

None of us is immune to disappointment or depression or fatigue or frustration. These feelings are a part of everyone's life at times. But becoming aware of the messages we send ourselves is the first step to pulling ourselves out of the quicksand of negative emotions.

Give it a try. The next time you catch yourself saying something negative about your situation, STOP. Perhaps you're running late for a parent-teacher meeting at school, and you get caught in traffic. You start to growl, "This is hopeless. I'm never going to get there, and even if I do, I'll be so late the teacher won't have time to tell me how my child is doing, and because of me, he'll probably fall behind and maybe not get promoted, and—"

STOP! Did you hear yourself just now? Because there were a few extra cars on the road and you weren't able to leave your office on time, you've just about delivered a failing grade to your wonderful kid, who works hard and does his best in school. You've given yourself a whopping dose of depression and anxiety, and you've tied your stomach in knots!

First, change the tone of your self-talk: "I'm not a victim. This is not the end of the world. If I'm too late, I'll ask the teacher to reschedule, or if we can speak on the phone. Now, what can I do while I'm waiting in this traffic? Why not make a list of my questions and concerns to refer to during the meeting? Or, hmm, maybe if I make a right at the next corner, I can get there faster by the back roads."

Second, remind yourself that you're doing the best you can under the circumstances. Just keep in mind that it's not what happens to us in life that determines how we live, but how we react and respond to it. You can't, at this moment, do anything much about the accident up ahead that's clogged the road. But you can at least not strangle yourself with guilt. And you can give yourself options for dealing with what happens next. Instead of being helpless and passive, you're still in charge of your life.

Almost every day I hear from people who have just about given up on themselves, who feel overwhelmed and tossed about by fate. I'll never forget a letter I received from a woman in Wisconsin who had suffered a terrible loss. Ellen's teenage daughter had died in a car accident, and she'd been numbing herself with food for months, dealing with her grief by eating at night instead of sleeping. She wrote after hearing me talk on QVC about my own feelings of helplessness and worthlessness, when my weight was so out of control and even my size-28 slacks were too tight. She'd begun going to support group meetings for parents who have lost children, and that, she said, was helping her cope with the flood of sorrow she still felt. And she'd started taking better care of herself and her husband, cooking healthier dishes from one of my cookbooks. But she wanted to know how I coped with the fear of losing control again, of letting the weight creep back on. She was slowly healing in both emotional and physical ways, but she still found herself listening to those old negative "tapes" that played and replayed in her memory.

So many people bring up this concern, and I always respond with what I learned through a long journey with lots of trial and error: that it's not about being in control, but about making choices—what to eat, what to do, how to live. Before I was able to figure this out for myself, I always felt out of control and helpless when it came to making healthy food choices. When a crash diet left me discouraged, depressed, and in even poorer health, I always blamed myself for my failure to do "whatever" long enough to lose my fanny. I couldn't acknowledge that the diet had held out false hope.

But finally I accepted the reality that there is no quick fix for our problems, whether they involve overeating, regulating blood sugar or cholesterol, or exercising to fight osteoporosis! Longlasting healthy-living practices take time to develop, and even more time to become habits. But by making the effort and working at these new behaviors, we discover a wonderful truth: that our hard work is the key to success. Instead of feeling victimized by everything from a plentiful buffet to a chronic medical condition, we've got the power to take care of ourselves!

Of course, it's important to make these lifestyle changes for the right reasons. It's one thing to do something because you *want* to please your partner, but it's quite another when you *have* to. If you want to lose a few pounds (or a few more than a few) so you'll feel better, then you're losing the weight for yourself.

But if your husband tells you that he won't be seen with you in public until you lose enough weight to wear a particular dress he likes, then he's making your weight loss a condition of his affection. You might struggle and lose enough weight to wear the dress once or twice, but it's unlikely that you'll be able to keep the weight off permanently.

People often share such concerns with me, especially when they've been hurt by things their loved ones have said to them. Most of the time, I hear from women who say, "My husband isn't happy with me because I've put on so much weight since we got married," or "He doesn't want to take me to the company party because he's embarrassed by how I look." Occasionally a man will share a similar comment, but more often it's women who pay the heavy price for our "shape-obsessed society."

I've been on both sides of the weight-loss issue in marriage, so I understand how confused and upset a woman can feel. When it came to my weight, nothing I *did* pleased my first husband. And nothing I *didn't* do disturbed my second.

When I was a bride back in 1966, I proudly designed and stitched my own wedding dress in a size 10/12. But within days of saying "I do," my groom began complaining that I was too fat and too tall. I allowed myself to become a victim of his demands. I desperately tried to please him by starving, slumping my shoulders, and wearing flats. But whenever I managed to lose a few pounds, it was never good enough. I eventually became a "closet eater" and ate almost nothing when he was around. But boy did I make up for it when I was alone! My weight fluctuated monthly, and my moods along with it. Sadly, the marriage didn't last, even though I forced myself to lose weight again just before we filed for divorce. I look back now with sadness, realizing that his own low self-esteem was bolstered only when he succeeded in destroying mine.

During the time it took for the divorce to become final, I

reacted to the stress and sorrow by turning to food. I managed to gain more than fifty pounds in just three months. I didn't even realize what I had done until I reached into my closet one day and discovered that nothing would fit me.

Later, when I met Cliff, my weight was at a *then* all-time high, but he thought I looked great anyway. I reacted by telling myself, "This man wants something and he's not going to get it." I gained another twenty pounds while we were dating. I understand now that subconsciously I was testing him to see if my weight would drive him away. It never did. He just kept calling me "his good-looking blonde" and asked me to marry him. In the eleven years we were married *before* I started living life in the Healthy Exchanges way, he never made an unkind comment about my weight. He saw me go on and off diets dozens of times and told me it wasn't necessary, because he loved me as I was and just wanted me to be happy with myself.

Nothing like finding a man like that to teach a woman who'd learned to be a victim not to be one anymore! It's been a decade or so since I changed my goal from losing weight to recapturing my health, and Cliff still calls me his "good-looking blonde!" He loved me *for me* when I wore size 20 in 1979 when we were married; he loved me *for me* when I wore a size 28 back in 1991, after twenty-eight years as a professional dieter; and he still loves me *for me* today as I happily wear a size 14. Sure, he's pleased with the new outer me, but *because I'm pleased*.

When we act helpless in the face of our problems, whether we're confronting a traffic jam or a hundred extra pounds, we're allowing ourselves to be victims, people who have no choice but to be shoved around by fate. By trying to change ourselves to fit someone else's idea of who we should be, we're surrendering the power that should be ours alone, and that's no good when it comes to making important decisions about our lives, our health, and our beliefs.

If you try to make changes in your life because someone else wants you to, or because a spouse gives you no choice in the matter, then your struggle for health and happiness comes with conditions. But lifestyle changes have the best shot of becoming permanent when you've got unconditional support and acceptance—and that begins with you. Until you accept and love yourself for the person you are *at this moment,* you're still vulnerable to victimhood. But once you begin to make changes for all the right reasons and in the right frame of mind, you've got the best possible chance to find the happiness and health you desire.

### A Pearl to Polish

*If for the next month, no one in your life put any pressure on you to lose weight, cut back on rich foods, or fit in some moderate exercise, would you still want to do it? And if you wanted to, what steps would you take to pursue your chosen path? Remember, no one is watching, commenting, or judging you. How does it feel to be the only one who decides whether you will do anything to improve your health or lower your stress level? I hope it feels good. I want you to try to remember that feeling. If you do decide to do something good for you,* do it for yourself, *and you'll know the joy of "no more being a victim!"*

# Resting on Your Laurels

*If you run into a wall, don't turn around and give up. Figure out how to climb it, go through it, or work around it.*

—MICHAEL JORDAN

*I* have no idea who first made the distinction between seeing a glass as half full or half empty, but I've always counted myself among those who tend to see and rejoice over what they have, not what they don't have. If my glass (or my plate) is half full, well, hurray, I still have half of my tasty main dish or delectable dessert left to eat. I wouldn't waste a second bemoaning the fact that I've already swallowed the first half of my portion. Doesn't that make sense to you?

I believe in applying a similar philosophy to the precarious time in a weight-loss or lifestyle-change program we call the Plateau. Most people find it a frustrating, heartbreaking, horrifying development—and they'll do just about anything to avoid it. Like what? you may ask. Oh, go on a starvation diet, consume nothing but liquids for a week, exercise for two hours a day, eat only cabbage soup or bananas until they turn green or yellow!

Is that any way to live? I don't think so.

But many people have confided in me that they feel like failures because they lost some weight and then they couldn't seem to lose another pound *no matter what they did!* Because they still have more to lose, and they're not losing even while doing what worked before, they think they must have done something WRONG. They ask me, in desperation, what to do, why they just can't seem to get "with it" anymore. They plead that time is passing and they've just got to get to their ideal weight, that perfect number, by next week, next month, as soon as possible.

Even if it took years of food abuse, of overeating and not being active, to get to this point, they're still impatient, frustrated, and even bitter. "I'm doing everything right, JoAnna," they say, "so why am I stuck?"

We've all lived so long in a society determined to enjoy instant gratification that if we can't get what we want right away, we are willing to do anything, no matter how unhealthy or outrageous, to get what we want NOW.

My philosophy about weight loss plateaus is that they're actually God's gift to your body (that is, as long as you truly are doing your part—eating healthy, exercising moderately, and thinking positively). Now why do I think something so radical and surprising? Even the most avid mountain climber won't take on Everest at a sprint. The stops along the way serve a real purpose, whether it's to help the body acclimatize to the altitude or simply to rest and replenish.

The journey to good health and permanent weight loss is basically the same. Most of us need to rest at a plateau now and then. This allows both our bodies and our minds to stabilize our weight loss. While we're resting "on our laurels" (what we've accomplished so far), what else might be happening? Well, for one, your skin has the opportunity to shrink along with your waist, so you don't start to look like "death warmed over" in the process. You can also use the extra time to let your mind catch up with your body. You've become a physically smaller person, but have you stopped thinking the way you did when you began to follow your healthy lifestyle plan? You may have gone from a size 20 to a size 12, but is your head still in the "large size" department? Or maybe your slacks are waist size 34 instead 40, but do you still gravitate to stretchy fabrics instead of selecting more fitted clothing?

A plateau is a time to focus on thinking and acting like the thinner, healthier person you are. Even if you've never been someone who can operate on "automatic pilot" when it comes to food, the way normally slender friends and family members might be able to, you can still train yourself to make conscious healthy decisions on a daily basis. When your attitude is "Hurry, hurry, rush, rush" to get down to your weight goal, you may not be thinking about the long term, only the time required to lose the weight. If you don't recognize that the changes you've made are best followed for a lifetime, you're at real risk of gaining the weight back and more!

I know from years of experience that when I was in a hurry, when I went rushing forward willing to do anything to see the needle on the scale move down, I never managed to sustain long-term or permanent weight loss. Arriving at a weight-loss goal was just a stop (and never a particularly long one) in a cycle of dieting and gaining, dieting and gaining, accompanied by guilt, shame, depression, or a sense of hopelessness. So when I decided to change my goal from simply losing weight to recapturing my health once and for all, I decided to change my attitude about the "dreaded" plateau too!

Most of us can do *anything* for the duration of a diet, because we know we don't have to do it for always. Trouble is, when we return to old habits, we get the same disappointing results—and we feel helpless in the face of such discouragement. But when we use the time of the plateau to strengthen our commitment to the changes we've made, we can feel much more confident that our good habits have replaced the old bad ones.

I've visited with so many people who have experienced plateaus on their journeys to permanent weight loss, and I've urged them not to use the temporary halt by the scale as an excuse to give up on themselves, or to change what they were doing for something less healthy and possibly faster in the short term. When it happened to me (and it happened more than once!), I kept measuring myself weekly to see what other changes had occurred in my body. I paid attention to how I felt when I exercised—did I have more bounce in my step? could I dance longer without taking a break? was I pedaling faster on my way to town on my bike? The evidence was there, but I had to make a point of looking for it. That, too, is one of the changes you need to make—focusing on the positive in a situation that has produced negative feelings in the past.

Even when the scale isn't providing a motivating "reward,"

people with a positive attitude look for other ways to feel good about themselves. Trying on a pair of jeans that you haven't worn in years, and managing to zip them up without holding your breath—isn't that even more exciting than seeing a half-pound lost on the scale? How about catching a glimpse of yourself in a store window and liking what you see? Compliments from friends who haven't seen you in a while have got to be worth some of the thrill of seeing the scale move steadily down—and if you don't feel that way now, act as if you do and you may soon find your attitude changing for the better.

If you're currently on a plateau, or if you're close to your goal but have another five to ten pounds you'd like to lose, try thinking about things in a new way. What if it takes six months, a year, or even more to lose those last unwanted pounds? At least you're not regaining any of what you've already lost. Instead of focusing on doing *anything* (including crash diets) to get those last pounds off, work on cementing your lost pounds into a permanent weight loss!

A plateau is a great time to reflect on what you've been doing, eating, thinking, and feeling. It's a good time to notice whether you've been in a food rut, eating the same few dishes every week, choosing the same three kinds of fruit at the market, always snacking on the same item each day at 4 P.M. When you get into a rut, sometimes your body does too, and so making a special effort to change what you're eating may trigger movement on the scale. If you've gotten a little lazy about cutting up vegetables or making fresh salads, focus on changing that, or at least buying some prepackaged ones to bolster whatever you've been eating lately.

What about activity? Have you stopped varying your exercise "diet," and instead walk the same couple of miles along the same route every day or two? It's still good exercise, don't get me wrong, but your body might sit up and take notice if you added a half hour of dancing to lively music once or twice a week! (So might your spouse and/or your kids!) Or if a friend has offered you guest passes to her health club, choose a day when you're getting your hair done the next, and jump in that swimming pool without caring a lick whether you get drenched or not!

I like to think of a plateau as a chance to renew, regroup, and refresh—the new three *R*s. First, it's a great time to **renew** your commitment to your healthy-living program. What do I mean by that? Read through your list of foods and find something new to try. Pick out a few new healthy recipes that intrigue you and maybe buy some new freezer containers if you can't find enough tops for the ones you have. If you've been eating a lot of dishes made with lean ground beef, give chicken breasts another try (at least occasionally). Why not stock up on healthy soups the next time the store has a special, so you'll be all set to prepare something on the spur of the moment? In fact, maybe this is a good time to renew your kitchen too, by tossing out old jars of spices and replacing them with fresh ones. Even if it's not time for spring cleaning, you could try "spring cleaning" your daily schedule: if you usually exercise in the morning, try an after-dinner walk with a friend for a change. If you always wear sweatpants and a sweatshirt when you work out, live "dangerously" and pick out a pair of exercise tights. They keep your legs warm, make you feel lean and fit, and if they've got enough Lycra in 'em, you'll look as sharp as you feel!

Now it's time to **regroup.** In a military situation, it would mean gathering the troops for a fresh onslaught on a target. In football, it's time for a huddle before the next play. For you, regrouping can mean gathering your resources for the next "push" forward. What resources might that include? Start with people. Would you enjoy finding an exercise buddy or adding a class to your schedule, just for a change? Do the research, ask around, get input from friends and colleagues at work. Then do something about it instead of just thinking it would be a good idea. What other roles might people play in your efforts? Are you a mother of young children who struggles to find time for herself? Maybe you need to organize an exercise co-op, where a group of moms work out together while splitting the cost of a baby-sitter. Are you a senior on a tight budget who would love to save more on healthy groceries but can't store those big multipacks from the discount clubs? Why not organize a shopping circle whose members take turns buying in quantity, sharing the cost, and divvying up the goods? Even if you're single, remember you're not alone!

Finally, use this time to take a pause to **refresh.** Have you been writing in a Positive Attitude journal recently? If not, would it help you to start again, at least for a while, to count your blessings and pat yourself on the back for all that you've accomplished. *Do it!*

This is a good time to reflect on your goals, the ones you set so long ago. Maybe they've changed a bit, and it's worthwhile to recognize that. Maybe you're ready to carve out some new ones that didn't even seem possible "way back when." Maybe you haven't rewarded yourself lately and you're overdue for a special nonfood treat?

Part of this pause to refresh should be philosophical. Remind yourself that no time is wasted, that while not every week produces weight loss or even an obvious physical change, every day still offers the wonderful possibility of growth and change deep within you. Think of how babies seem to change every day when they're young, and how joyfully each new accomplishment is heralded by those who love that child. When do we stop acknowledging with that same pleasure and even astonishment how we as human beings continue to evolve and transform ourselves? We learn a new skill on the computer at work, and yet no one applauds. Why is that, I wonder? Well, maybe the only one who will clap hands on your behalf is you, but you still deserve it. When you finally understand what your broker is talking about when he says you should consider investing in an IPO, congratulations! When you at last find a hair product to tame that cowlick that has tormented you for months, good for you! All those little things are pluses, and you'll be pleased at how powerfully refreshed you'll feel when you start crediting your personal account with those self-esteem "dollars."

I can't even begin to explain the thrill of reaching into my closet for clothes that still fit from last year—or are even a bit too big to wear. I never got to enjoy that in my life as a professional dieter. I never knew whether I'd be heavier or thinner from year to year. But because I allowed my body to call the shots, I don't think I look like a middle-aged woman who has lost more weight than many slender women weigh! I like what I see in my mirror, and I felt such pride on my birthday this year when I reflected for a moment on how I turned my life around, even if it took almost a half century to do it!

Now, see, you thought a time of plateauing was a time of sitting still, getting frustrated, being STUCK. Instead, I'm suggesting that it's not an obscene word, but a great opportunity to take all kinds of action to keep yourself going in the direction of your dreams.

### A Pearl to Polish

*If you're experiencing a plateau in your weight-loss efforts, start by checking up on what you're doing daily, and determine that you're truly doing your part to get there. If you are, remind your body to do its part, and then turn your attention elsewhere. Instead of weighing yourself down with fear and discouragement, relax your shoulders, lift your head, and tackle any one of the Three Rs—renew, regroup, refresh. Sometimes even the smallest change is enough to kick-start your efforts; other times, it'll take all the patience you can muster to get the scale going down again. But since you're not standing still in other ways that matter, it's a lot easier to feel you're going somewhere.*

# Why Now Is the Best Time

*It's a job that's never started that takes the longest to finish.*

—J. R. R. TOLKIEN

*I* discovered author Barbara Sher years ago, when she wrote a wonderfully motivating book called *Wishcraft,* which gave all kinds of help in figuring out what you most wanted in life and how to go after it. Recently, she published *It's Only Too Late If You Don't Start Now,* a book whose title so inspired me, I began writing this chapter after spotting it on a bookstore shelf.

I love this title because it's so often a topic that comes up when people visit with me. "It's too late," they say. "I've been eating this way for so long, I don't think I can change." Or perhaps someone will murmur in a discouraged voice, "Now that I'm over fifty and in menopause, I lose weight so slowly that I can't stay motivated." Or maybe another will say, "Well, my daughter's wedding is only four months away, and I've got sixty pounds to lose, so I need something more drastic, something quicker—"

Time is one of the greatest gifts we have on this earth, time to spend with loved ones, time to raise children and stretch our minds and give back to the community. Giving time, making time, finding time—it's become a kind of obsession. But for too many people, time is an enemy, an obstacle that stands in the way of what we say we want. "I don't have time to exercise," one young woman told me recently. "I already get up at six to get ready for work, and by the time I get home from my job, it's dark out." She is defeated before she even starts. She's told herself something is impossible, and after a while comes to believe it's true. So for her I'd alter the "mantra" slightly: It's impossible only if you don't give it a try. I'm a very early riser, which I realize isn't for everyone, but I asked Melanie if she was a morning person or a night person. "Morning," she answered, and so I suggested she experiment with a slight change in her morning routine. I asked her to get up ten minutes earlier two or three times a week, lace on her sneakers, and walk around the street she lives on for fifteen minutes. I "snitched" five minutes from the time she already had set aside for getting ready for work. If she felt there was more room in her evening routine, I suggested she make her lunch the night before, lay out her clothes, and pack her briefcase in advance. Before long, she discovered she could stretch her morning walks into thirty minutes, and she began enjoying her quiet time so much that she tried to do it four to five times a week!

For so many people, time is a painful issue that influences how we approach all lifestyle changes. I remember speaking with

Annette, a woman in her forties who said she deeply regretted that she wasn't married, and who believed her need to lose a lot of weight was a major reason for the situation. She had just begun using my recipes and HELP plan and had lost about ten pounds so far. But instead of being excited and looking forward to the future, she was surprisingly melancholy. "If I do lose the weight now, I still may not meet someone, and if it turns out my weight wasn't the reason for not finding a husband, then what excuse can I give myself and my parents? And if I *do* meet someone, I'll always know that if only I'd done this sooner, I wouldn't have missed out on so much."

I wanted to give Annette a fresh perspective on her situation, especially since I didn't lose my weight for the last time until I was in my forties. I reminded her of my own story, and that I had married the true love of my life the second time around (so I believe there is good reason to be optimistic about finding love after the first glow of youth)!

But even more, I told her that the past is just that—past. She can't change it, she can't regret it, because the energy it takes to mourn what didn't happen in her life is wasted energy. And while it's important to set goals for the future, the present is all we've really got. What's important to me, and I believe, for all of us, is to focus on what we *can* do about where we are now.

I suggested that Annette devote her attention to the good in her life right now. "You've begun eating healthy, and it's paying off with real results. Keep up the good work, and beware of falling back into a dieting mentality. Eat what you like in my healthy versions, and get out of the house. You may meet a wonderful guy or you may not, but in the meantime, it's important to stay active, get involved in activities you enjoy, and put some energy into the world outside yourself." She had always loved ballroom dancing but hadn't danced in years because she felt that no one would want to dance with her heavier self. With my encouragement and her own determination, she signed up for a class at the community college near her home. She's continued her weight loss, she's polished her dancing technique beautifully, and while she hasn't met Mr. Right just yet, she's danced with lots of interesting men!

So many men and women find their way to me in later life, because that's when they're diagnosed with heart conditions, high blood pressure and cholesterol, or diabetes. Many of them are scared they won't be able to make the kinds of changes their doctors insist they must. One woman wrote to me that the doctor wanted her husband to follow a strict 1,400-calorie diabetic diet to lose weight, but that she refused to do it. "First," she wrote, "I knew we'd never stay on it. Second, he works sixty to eighty hours a week and would never survive on so few calories. And third, we needed something that we could follow for the rest of our lives." I'm pleased to note that she spotted my cookbooks at her local bookstore and began preparing healthy meals that made sense. In three months, her husband lost more than thirty pounds and she'd lost twenty-five! They recognized that a change was necessary, but needed realistic advice they could live with.

I often hear from women and men in their seventies and eighties who discover that it's never too late to start living healthy. Sometimes I want to hand their letters out to younger people who come up to me and say, "Oh, it's too late, I've been heavy all my life." Or to those who want a faster fix than I would ever promise them, saying, "It's too late, I've got to be thin before my high school reunion, so I'm going to try a liquid diet for a few weeks." They may experience some quick water-weight loss, but keeping those pounds off for very long is going to be difficult. I can tell them from my own experience!

Sometimes it's the notion of exercising that strikes people as too much to ask, especially when they're feeling creaky or can't make it up a flight of stairs. I've had lots of people tell me that they've never been athletic, so forget about going to the gym. Or, they add, they get breathless walking to the mailbox, and they're completely uncoordinated, so aerobics is out.

I don't give up so easily, they soon find out. Okay, I'll say, I want you to walk to the mailbox three times a day. Once in the morning, when you're sure the postman hasn't been there, but you just want to check. Later, when you're pretty certain the mail has arrived, to bring it in. And once again in the late afternoon, when you know there probably isn't any mail in the box, but you might have missed something. If you find yourself getting out of breath, then slow down, but keep doing it, and I promise that soon it will get easier.

I heard from one delightful woman who was eighty years young and determined to get that last ten pounds off no matter what. She knew without hearing it from me, or anyone else, that it *is too late only if you don't start now,* and she decided to stick with what was working. She wrote, "I'd decided that at my age I didn't want to cook anymore, but then I just had to try a couple of your desserts. From there I progressed to entrees—the food is so much better than TV dinners!"

What I love about Allie's attitude is that she isn't letting age stand in the way of her dreams of better health. Even a fractured hip didn't dissuade her from trying to live well, and the spirit and joy that sizzle off the page made me reexamine my own attitudes about what I can and can't do as I get older.

I've been confronting many changes in my own life the past few years—the "power surges" of menopause, the reaching of that age-fifty-five plateau where I get the senior discount at Hardee's. I've learned that every cycle and phase of life is different, but I'm also learning that each has its surprises and unexpected pleasures. Some things are not as easy as they once were, but I appreciate them more. I can't do everything in my fifties that I could do in my thirties, but there are many things I do now that I never imagined doing back then—speaking to large groups of people, writing books and newsletters, and appearing on television to share my message.

When you're thirty, you think you've got forever to do whatever you want to do. By fifty, though, you may begin to feel that life is passing you by. You're more concerned about health issues, you're coping with medical concerns you may never have imagined would affect you. So it's especially important to keep the positive attitude you had when you were younger and use it to shape your middle and later years.

I remember arguing with my ex-husband years ago about something I wanted to do. He kept giving me all kinds of negative responses—"Don't even try because you'll fail," or "Forget it—it's too late," or "What's the use?" I insisted that I'd never know until I tried, and that's been my philosophy for so many years now. I may not make all my dreams real, but I don't want anyone telling me I'm too old to do what I want, or that my time has passed. I'm determined not to believe it!

I always say that "now is the best time of all." Now is all we're certain of, and we need to take it more seriously. We spend so much of our lives planning for the future, saving for the future, living for the future, but if you put everything on hold, you may miss far too much of the joy of today.

So say it with me: It's not too late. It's never too late. It's only too late (thanks to Ms. Sher!) if you don't start now. Please take those dreams off hold and start walking in their direction. Make today the very best day you can—and start again tomorrow!

### A Pearl to Polish

*My sister Regina wrote this poem years ago when she was a teenager, and it seems a perfect way to end this chapter:*

### Time

*Time is progress.*
    *It never ceases.*
*When I am tired and rest, Time continues on.*
    *I must cherish Time—every precious moment of it.*
*When I have departed from this earth,*
    *Time will not stop because of me.*

*It will go onward, not even knowing or caring*
    *about me.*
*I must admire Time; I can only think how tired*
    *Time must be.*
*Never stopping to rest.*
    *For Time is Eternity.*

                    *—Regina McAndrews Reyes*

# If Your Best Is Good Enough for God, Let It Be Good Enough for You

*I come to the office each morning and stay for long hours doing what has to be done to the best of my ability. And when you've done the best you can, you can't do any better. So when I go to sleep, I turn everything over to the Lord and forget it.*

—HARRY S TRUMAN

My parents always taught me and my sisters that God expected us to do our best, whether we were doing homework or helping around the house, digging in the garden or practicing music or for a play at school. Getting good grades was important, of course, but the emphasis was on doing the best you could—and that didn't always mean getting straight A's.

I've tried to carry that philosophy into all parts of my adult life—at work, of course, and also at home as I raised my own children. I did my best to teach them to work hard and give their best efforts in everything they did. They grew to adulthood with good characters and with self-esteem that encouraged them to strive for difficult goals and achieve them. Now that they are parents themselves, I smile with pride as I see them teaching their children what I tried to teach them—that doing your best brings life's true rewards.

But doing your best means taking responsibility for your actions every day of your life. It means saying, "Yes, I did that, and I'm satisfied with the effort I made. I'd like to do better tomorrow, but for today, this is the best I could do."

The dictionary defines responsibility as, first, the condition or quality of being responsible; obligation; accountability; dependability; and, second, as a thing or person one is responsible for. Those definitions make demands that are not easily avoided, yet many people seem unprepared to accept responsibility in their everyday lives.

Some prefer to blame their ancestors for their "big bones" or thick waist, while at the same time they've been digging into bags of potato chips every night for a week. Some hope to push the blame for their elevated blood sugar onto family members who bring home boxes of donuts; others insist they've got no time for a brisk walk at night, yet can always be found seated in front of the television with a bag of cookies at the ready. Some have tired of the debate over whether butter or margarine is worse for your health, and are just soaking their bread in dishes of olive oil, forgetting that it's all just fat!

Isn't it about time that we take responsibility for our actions? I realize that it's not the most popular position to take, considering all the television shows devoted to blaming others for our problems or expecting others to solve them. Sometimes, as I flip through the channels, it seems that every one features people yelling at the top of their lungs that it's someone else's fault, crying that "if only" they'd been treated differently they'd never have ended up with such problems! Some of those "if only" excuses would almost be funny if they weren't so sad. But making excuses is the exact opposite of taking responsibility. As long as someone else can be blamed for a situation, people feel free to sit back and make no effort to make things better, because after all, "It's not my fault."

To be responsible means to be accountable to yourself. Let me say it another way: **You, and you alone, are responsible and accountable for your actions.** Some days it seems our country is falling apart at the seams simply because too few people are prepared to accept responsibility for their actions. Children go to class without their homework and insist the dog ate it (a golden oldie) or it fell behind the desk and they couldn't reach it. Teenagers who attend unsupervised parties where beer is available blame peer pressure for why they got drunk, when the truth is that they were unwilling to say no. Malpractice insurance rates keep rising, not because doctors are so much worse than they used to be, but because too many people want to use the legal system to place blame for a less-than-perfect medical outcome.

There's no point in focusing on the big picture when it comes to taking responsibility; it's enough to become accountable just to ourselves. By taking a good, hard look in our internal mirrors, we realize that no one forced us to gobble down the remaining six slices of cold pizza at midnight. We recognize that it's up to us, and only us, to find twenty minutes for a walk in an otherwise busy day. We start to accept that we can't do a thing about the past, but we can surely improve the future.

I know it can be scary to accept responsibility for what you've done up to this point. After all, for twenty-eight years, I blamed everyone and everything but my out-of-control eating and couch potato habits for my excess weight and health problems! It was easier to tell myself that I wasn't the cause of my troubles than to recognize that only I could make the changes that would transform my body and my life. And it was only when I faced the truth, that I was responsible for what and how much I put into my mouth, that I could learn to eat in moderation.

Blaming circumstances or other people is a little like living in a dictatorship—you persuade yourself that *you have no choice,* that things would be different if it were up to you. The thing is, of course, that it *is* up to you, and that it has almost always been in your hands. I'm not saying that you have complete control over every aspect of your life, because you may not, but you do have control over how you respond to each decision you're faced with and each crossroads you approach.

What changed for me when I finally accepted responsibility for my health and well-being is that I learned to make those decisions: to choose which foods I ate and how much, to organize my day to fit in some moderate exercise, and to recognize what elements of my life were contributing to my weight problems and ill health. For me, it meant developing self-discipline, and in the process I found a surprising satisfaction in making the decisions that helped me recapture my health and lose 130 pounds.

It didn't mean deprivation, which surprised me. Instead,

knowing I had the power to make choices let me enjoy what I chose in a way I never really had before. Instead of spicing my meals with guilt and shame, I could dine in confidence that I was eating for health and taking pleasure in every bite!

That's why MODERATION became the password to my new life, and why I believe it can help you achieve yours as well. By taking responsibility for what I ate, how I exercised, the goals I set, and the positive habits I developed, I felt finally free to live fully in the Real World. I practice self-discipline when I choose to eat realistic portions of healthy foods. I vowed never again to nibble on carrot sticks with a diet soda as a chaser and call it a meal. That's deprivation, and it only leads to misery and binge-ing. But I also promised myself I wasn't going to gobble down an entire cake or casserole and call it a snack! That's gluttony, and it only brings a sense of overwhelming shame and guilt that shatters self-esteem. Instead, I eat responsibly, enjoying moderate portions of a variety of foods, and relish my meals as I never have before.

By simply deciding to accept no more excuses from myself when it came to what I ate and how I lived, I not only recaptured my health but I reclaimed my commitment to do the best I can every day. By taking responsibility for what I did, I discovered a deeper connection with the Lord, because I felt that in His eyes, I was fulfilling what He wanted from me.

Are there days when I'm not satisfied with what I've managed to accomplish? Of course. I'm human, and fallible, and imperfect, just as we all are. I get impatient and frustrated with myself and others. But instead of sinking into the quicksand of negative thinking, which is certain to do me no good, I try to accept that today I did what I could, and tomorrow I will try to do better, aiming for the best I can do.

Do you feel that you have been making excuses for any of the problems or disappointments you may be facing in your own life? Have you been stuck in a kind of rut, hoping for a miracle of some kind that would make those difficulties vanish? Does the idea of striving to live your life better seem too exhausting or impossible to attempt?

It may be because your expectations are inflated beyond what makes sense for you at the moment. I'm not suggesting that you settle for goals far below what you want for yourself, but rather that getting where you want to go will take more time, faith, and patience than you expected. You may not see the kind of progress you would like for a while, but if you are moving, however slowly, toward those dreams you hold dear, then your daily best is more than good enough. One of my readers quoted Dr. George Sheehan, the running guru, on this subject. He said, "There are days when I can't get the ball in the basket, no matter how hard I try. But there is no excuse for not playing good defense." For the less sports-minded (and I count myself among you!), he's referring to giving your best effort without being focused only on the measurable results. Maybe you scored no points in the basketball game of life today, but if you ran your heart out and played the best you could, then you earned your place on the team.

God never asks you to do more than you can, so when the burden feels like more than you can bear, remember that God is just a prayer away.

## *A Pearl to Polish*

*Sometimes, the responsibility of doing what you believe is your best is overwhelming, and you feel like buckling under the weight of expectations, even if they are only the ones you have for yourself. Perhaps you will be able to dig deeper on another one; possibly, you will be more inspired, more understanding, more energetic tomorrow or next week. All you can do today is give it your best effort, and know that the Lord sees that you have. Instead of wallowing in negativity or focusing on what you were unable to achieve on a given day, accept your effort and rest easier at night, knowing that tomorrow will present a new opportunity to reach for the best you can be.*

# I want to hear from you . . .

I've given you a road map in *String of Pearls,* and I hope it will help you reach for your dreams. But if you ever find you're stumbling on your personal journey toward self-acceptance and good health, you can always check in with me. Write to:

JoAnna M. Lund
c/o Healthy Exchanges, Inc.
PO Box 124
DeWitt, IA 52742

Or, if you prefer, you can fax me at 1-319-659-2126 or contact me via e-mail by writing to HealthyJo@aol.com. And please visit my Healthy Exchanges Internet website at: http://www. healthyexchanges.com. You'll find support and friendship on our message boards and in the chat room.